The International Behavioural and Social Sciences Library

COMMUNICATIONS IN THE BUILDING INDUSTRY

TAVISTOCK

The International Behavioural and Social Sciences Library

INDUSTRIAL RELATIONS
In 13 Volumes

I	Efficiency and Effort *W Baldamus*
II	Interdependence and Uncertainty *Edited by Charles Crichton*
III	Form and Content in Industrial Democracy *F E Emery and Einar Thorsrud*
IV	The Dynamics of a Changing Technology *Peter J Fensham and Douglas Hooper*
V	Communications in the Building Industry *Gurth Higgin and Neil Jessop*
VI	The Game of Budget Control *G H Hofstede*
VII	The Changing Culture of a Factory *Elliott Jaques*
VIII	Measurement of Responsibility *Elliott Jaques*
IX	Mid-Career Development *Robert N Rapoport*
X	The Enterprise and its Environment *A K Rice*
XI	Managers *Kenn Rogers*
XII	New Ways in Management Training *Cyril Sofer and Geoffrey Hutton*
XIII	The Enterprise in Transition *H van der Haas*

COMMUNICATIONS IN THE BUILDING INDUSTRY

The Report of a Pilot Study

GURTH HIGGIN AND NEIL JESSOP

ROUTLEDGE
Taylor & Francis Group

First published in 1965 by
Tavistock Publications Limited

Reprinted in 2001 by
Routledge
2 Park Square, Milton Park, Abingdon, Oxon, OX14 4RN
270 Madison Ave, New York NY 10016

Transferred to Digital Printing 2008

Routledge is an imprint of the Taylor & Francis Group

British Library Cataloguing in Publication Data
A CIP catalogue record for this book
is available from the British Library

Communications in the Building Industry
ISBN 0-415-26440-5
Industrial Relations: 13 Volumes
ISBN 0-415-26510-X
The International Behavioural and Social Sciences Library
112 Volumes
ISBN 0-415-25670-4

ISBN10: 0–415–26440–5 (hbk)
ISBN10: 0–415–48415–4 (pbk)

ISBN13: 978–0–415–26440–2 (hbk)
ISBN13: 978–0–415–48415–2 (pbk)

Communications in the Building Industry

THE REPORT OF A PILOT STUDY

GURTH HIGGIN

The Committee on Human Resources, Organisation and Social Change

& NEIL JESSOP

Director, The Institute for Operational Research

Of The Tavistock Institute of Human Relations

TAVISTOCK PUBLICATIONS

First published by Tavistock Publications 1965

Printed in Great Britain by Compton Printing Works (London) Ltd

CONTENTS

PART TWO

PROBLEMS, RECOMMENDATIONS, AND REQUIREMENTS

APPENDICES

PREFACE TO THE SECOND EDITION

To refer to this pamphlet as a second edition is something of a misnomer. More accurately it is the first general publication of a working paper reporting a three months' pilot study, undertaken by the Tavistock Institute of Human Relations, which was commissioned by the National Joint Consultative Committee of Architects, Quantity Surveyors and Builders under my predecessor, Sir William Holford. As the conclusions of the study went beyond the concerns of the members of the National Joint Consultative Committee, a conference representative of all interests in the Building Industry was called by the Committee to receive and consider the report.

The conference endorsed the approach exemplified in the Pilot Study as of value to the Industry, and unanimously agreed to support continuance of research along these lines. With this encouragement the National Joint Consultative Committee invited others, including the Ministry of Public Building and Works and the Department of Scientific and Industrial Research, to join with it in setting up a body that would sponsor further research of this kind on behalf of the Building Industry as a whole. This became the Building Industry Communications Research Committee, for which Lord James of Rusholme agreed to become the independent chairman. In an epilogue Lord James briefly records developments since responsibility for this work passed from the National Joint Consultative Committee.

Although the report was widely distributed in a duplicated version at the time of the original conference, there has been a steady, and recently increasing, demand for copies - hence the decision to publish it in this present form.

Being only a pilot study, and produced in a very limited time, the report did not claim to be a comprehensive or definitive statement about the Industry. The emphasis it gives design, for example, is rather less than does justice to its place in the building process, and the importance of the contributions of engineering consultants, suppliers merchants and sub-contractors are not fully dealt with. Nevertheless, the conference which received it did not consider these points detracted from the value of the analysis presented. The authors have consequently not attempted to re-write the report. Apart from the correction of a few minor errors of fact, it is offered here in its original form.

J. G. OSBORNE
CHAIRMAN

National Joint Consultative Committee of Architects, Quantity Surveyors & Builders

December 1964

FOREWORD

This document reports the results of our three months' study of the building industry and our reflections on what we have learned.

It is in two parts. Part One we have called a Field Report. This presents a picture of the industry as reflected by a Sociological/ Operational Research mirror. The picture is not complete, it may be blurred in places, and there are almost certainly some distortions in it. We hope, nevertheless, that its general outlines are recognisable to those who know the original better than we do.

Part Two is a summary of the general conclusions we have arrived at, and recommends what we consider the disciplines we represent could offer to the industry by way of research. Part Two opens with a list of what we see as the main questions associated with communications in the industry. We next provide a very condensed version of our main thesis, about what lies behind the industry's communications difficulties, by way of preamble to a three-part research recommendation. We then discuss the conditions necessary for the industry to embark on this sort of research, and make two further recommendations about the requirements for launching it.

At this time we would like to express our thanks to all those in the industry and associated with it who have been so helpful to us in our enquiries. Everybody we have approached has given us unstinted time and attention. We have also been struck by the intense interest our study has universally produced. This has been a great encouragement to us, and, we feel, is a promising sign for the future of the industry.

PART ONE

A FIELD REPORT

SECTION I

INTRODUCTION

The Background of the Project

1. At its meeting on the 12th October 1962, The National Joint Consultative Committee decided, after considering a report from a sub-committee on "Communications in the Building Industry":

> "that a pilot study lasting about three months should start not later than December 1st and should report to a conference representative of the industry to be arranged at a Cambridge College during the Easter Vacation 1963."

2. As we understand it, the process leading up to this decision started with a resolution at the 1961 Annual General Meeting of the South Western Federation of Building Trade Employers, which recommended that: "Annotated Bills of Quantities are a necessity". This resolution was passed to the South Western Joint Consultative Committee who in turn passed it on to the National Joint Consultative Committee, the Administrative Committee of which body considered the resolution on the 15th March 1962. In the report of this meeting it is stated that:

> "discussion by the Administrative Committee showed that this was really only one facet of the general problems of communication in the Building Industry which was engaging the attention of all three constituent bodies in different ways. It was felt co-ordination in this field might usefully be discussed by the NJCC at the annual conference."

3. The Administrative Committee set up a sub-committee of three to consider this question. This sub-committee reported to the Annual Conference of Regional Consultative Committee Chairmen and Secretaries in May 1962. This sub-committee noted the reaction, particularly from the RICS, against a move to make annotated bills compulsory. It considered that this was part of a wider question, which was expressed as "How simply and completely can the needs of the building authority be identified, interpreted, notified and transmitted to those who have to submit offers and in due course execute building work?" It further reported that:

"dissatisfaction with the present system of communication between members of the building team is widespread. It is reflected in Builders' demands for 'full documentation' at the time of tendering; the Architects' difficulties in using Consultants' services effectively, and the development of new forms of Bill and new methods of measurement by Surveyors... The survey of the problems facing the construction industry recently prepared for the Minister of Works by Sir Harold Emmerson, has emphasised the lack of cohesion between the Architect and his professional colleagues and the Builder, and this is in large part the result of faulty systems of communication... The NJCC felt there was need here ... for a general examination of the whole problem to see where additional study was needed and how it best could be undertaken."

4. The conference discussed the sub-committee's report very fully and passed it back to the NJCC for further consideration, and if thought necessary, action.

5. The NJCC requested the sub-committee to continue with their task, and to suggest what action it should take in view of the suggestions made at the annual conference that what was required now was some form of research rather than a continuation of discussion.

6. Initially the sub-committee thought of the possibility of setting up some fairly long term fundamental research on the general problem. On further examination they decided that the question of communications in the building industry was too complex even to be able to state clear research problems at this stage and that a study to clarify the problem was a necessary first step. A detailed record of the considerations that led the sub-committee from this point to the NJCC resolution reported above is given in Appendix A and its attachments.

7. To take charge of the research project on their behalf, the NJCC appointed a steering committee made up of the three original members of the sub-committee with four additions. In early meetings with the steering committee the attention of the research team was drawn to the statement in the Emmerson Report concerning the need for co-operation and cohesion in the building industry, and they were asked to bear in mind that improvements in communications should be thought of as serving this general objective.

SECTION II

THE TECHNIQUES OF COMMUNICATION AND THEIR USES

1. In this section we will describe the picture that we have built up of the principal forms of communication in the building process* and how they are used. As will be seen from our account below the subject is one of considerable variety, even of confusion. For the purposes of this exposition we have divided the building process up into seven phases, set out in the following table.

Phases of the Building Process

Phase 0.	Client deciding to build.
Phase 1.	Client consulting building team sponsor.
Phase 2.	Sponsor investigating and preparing the brief.
Phase 3.	Preparing and gaining client's acceptance for sketch plans. Obtaining outline approvals.
Phase 4.	Preparing contract documents. Obtaining final approvals.
Phase 5.	Preparing and agreeing contract. Setting up construction team.
Phase 6.	Construction to completion.
Phase 7.	Handing over and settling final account.

2. In what follows a distinction is made between formal and informal techniques of communication. Formal communications are simply those that have some concrete form and provide a record. In general this is anything that is on paper whether it is in the form of words, drawings or numbers. Informal techniques are those that do not automatically leave a record. This category includes oral communication and what we refer to as trivia. Oral communications may be pre-arranged discussions, casual conversations, or telephone calls. Trivia covers such things as scribbles on the back of an envelope, a sketch on the back of a menu or a calculation on a

---

* All that happens in the process which starts with a client's need and ends with the delivery of a finished structure designed to satisfy this need.

tablecloth. In some cases the communication carried by a trivial technique is confirmed in formal form later. We include trivia not to suggest that the building industry is unique in communicating in this way, but because we have been struck by the number of examples we have met in which quite crucial pieces of information essential to important decisions have been made in this way.

3. Under the headings in this section we will say something of the techniques we have found to be used typically for each phase, something of the factors which seem to affect their use, together with comments on these points.

Phase 0. Client Deciding to Build

4. The decisions made by a client during this phase will determine the sorts of approaches that will be made to members of the building industry when the next phase is reached. In considering this we distinguish between the levels of sophistication of clients. By the sophisticated client we mean a person or an organisation who knows a good deal, usually from experience, about the building process and of the contributions of the various members of a building team. Typical examples are the developer who embodies a wide, if not full, range of building team skills in his own organisation, and the large public authority for whom the same thing is true. These are sophisticated clients who are well served with advice at this stage. At the other end of the scale is the naive client, the organisation which has not built before, or not for some time, or the individual who knows little or nothing of building. In the process of reaching a decision to build the naive client will usually seek some sort of advice or attempt to get some relevant information before reaching his final decision. This however is an initial move that he must make from almost complete ignorance. His first adviser may be another client of greater sophistication than himself. Whatever his decision is it will have an important effect upon the nature of the building team that will follow and upon the pattern of communications it will develop.

5. Various organisations involved in building have attempted to communicate with the prospective clients of the industry, in particular the RIBA, through articles and leaflets. In the main however it would seem to be personal contact that decides the naive client's decision.

Phase 1. Client Consulting Building Team Sponsor

6. We define sponsor as the member of the team first approached by the client, who is thus put in the position of, if not inviting, at least advising on invitations to further members of the team. The use of the term is described more fully in the second attachment to Appendix A.

7. The first communication from client to sponsor may be a letter, or an oral or telephone enquiry, followed by a meeting. If the process continues from that point, formal communications, letters, memoranda etc., and, within a short space, sketches, designs and cost information will quickly follow.

8. As to who is involved and for what purpose, we have found this to be variable. The traditional first contact and sponsor of the building team is the architect. This however would not seem to be a universal practice, particularly with sophisticated clients. We have met cases where quantity surveyors and builders have been put in the sponsor role. This choice would seem to be determined by the nature of the client's building need. The developer, for example, whose interest in building is basically commercial, tends to make his first approach to a quantity surveyor who specialises in cost estimating. Other more naive clients who know only the traditional custom, and those more interested in design or function, tend to approach an architect. Builders seem to be approached for either historical or technical reasons. By historical reasons we mean, for example, a large industrial organisation with many scattered installations which is always engaged in building of some kind, if not new building then extension and repair. Such an organisation may have a quasi-permanent relationship with a building firm which, it is understood by both parties, will undertake any new building for the organisation. Thus when a decision is made to put up a new building the organisation will approach this builder in the first instance. The builder will advise on the choice of the other members of the team. The technical reason for approaching a builder is the interest of a client in some particular building system or technique in which that builder specialises. This information may have been communicated to him, perhaps informally, by any other person, or through the technical or general press. In this latter case, of course, he has been using the press as a means of communication in taking his decision under the previous phase.

9. There is also the role of internal sponsor - the architect or surveyor (often a valuation surveyor) inside the client organisation. Such an organisation may have as its main function a continuous interest in building - a developer for instance, or the housing committee of a public authority. In such cases the internal sponsor will be activated by a formal instruction, although the reverse could also hold. That is, the internal sponsor informs his principals that conditions in respect to money, availability of land or planning approvals are now favourable to action.

Phase 2. Sponsor Investigating and Preparing the Brief

10. In our short acquaintance with the industry we have found that this phase covers a tremendous variety of techniques of communication and we can well believe that there is non that has not, at some time, been used in this phase of the building process. There is a long list of formal and more usual techniques involved - letters, memoranda, questionnaires, check lists, models, photographs of buildings and photographs of models, and perspective drawings, plain or coloured. In addition to these formal techniques, in investigating and brief-building there is a high proportion of informal techniques involved - talking, telephoning, trivia, the passing of books and journals etc.

11. We have also been surprised at the long list of the sorts of people with whom these communications, usually of a consulting nature, will be undertaken - chemists, physicists, engineers of all kinds, doctors, financiers, sociologists, other clients, meteorologists, and many others.

12. To ensure the ideal result from this phase of the process it is understandable that the range of resources and techniques of communication called upon needs to be comprehensive. If the study of a client's needs - financial, aesthetic, functional and social - is to be complete, the sponsor will have to know the needs of the client very intimately, whether an individual or an organisation. He will also need to undertake a similar thorough study of relevant building resources to ensure that the best possible solutions to the client's needs are found. The sponsor, no matter what his particular expertise, will obviously need assistance if this dual task is to be performed adequately. Even the architect, the man whom one would expect to be best qualified to undertake it, is unlikely to command sufficient

knowledge, particularly in the fields of technology and costing, to be able to do it all himself. We suspect that this very important phase of the building process is at times not done adequately because the original sponsor has not realised, or is not willing to accept, the need for the application of a wider knowledge than he himself can easily command. This situation can give rise to difficulties, particularly at later stages of the building process when undiscovered needs or unexplored solutions appear. Even if the investigation is adequate, equally serious difficulties can arise if enough trouble is not taken at this time to ensure that the brief which embodies it is the subject of full understanding and agreement by all parties. This is particularly the case in respect of the often vexed question of expenditure.

13. For a client who is not sophisticated in the sense in which we are using that term, it is not easy to define and communicate his needs. This is particularly true when the client is a corporate public body. The reaction of the architect, the man usually responsible for working with the client on this job, tends to be one of frustration and impatience, largely, we suspect, from a sense of inability to help. There is often very real and unavoidable confusion for a naive client in exploring and reconciling conflicting internal needs. There are techniques for assisting this type of process in the social sciences (problem identification, conflict resolution etc.) as well as within the industry (59), which we would suggest should be better known and employed by architects. Given greater understanding and tolerance by the architect of the client's confusion, and some tools for helping him, the task of preparing a brief might be done more expeditiously and more effectively. We know of one case where these conditions applied, leading to a very satisfactory outcome. This case has also been publicly reported (23).

14. It is at this point in the building process that the possibility of a conflict of values within the building team can first show itself. If, as is usually the case, there are several members of the building team sharing the work of constructing the brief, any one of them, but particularly the one in the role of sponsor, can unbalance the whole by a too single-minded pursuit of perfection for those aspects that are his especial concern. The architect/sponsor, for example, will be tempted to maximise architectural magnificence at the expense of time, cost, or technological considerations, the quantity surveyor/sponsor to maximise economy at the expense of architectural or technological considerations, and the builder/sponsor to maximise profit at the expense of architecture and client's

financial outlay. Many of the communications which pass at this time between the parties involved, including the client, arise from the development of these conflicts and the need to resolve them. This is a process of optimisation, a process which arises continually in the building process and to which we shall return several times in our report.

Phase 3. Preparing and Gaining Client's Acceptance for Sketch Plans Obtaining Outline Approvals

15. If the previous phase can be thought of as the search for strategic decisions for the forthcoming building operation, this phase can be thought of as the search for tactical decisions. Its starting point is the strategic decisions arrived at in the previous phase and embodied in the brief. To develop the tactics from these strategic decisions the team involved needs to be enlarged. Thus early communications in this phase take the form of invitations to others to join the emerging building team. These further people tend to be in specialist roles. They may be consultants in the various fields of engineering, or contractors in these fields who also undertake design, or they can be specialist manufacturers who also design.

16. These invitations may take the form of a request for advice on a small contained problem, an offer of participation in the design process, an offer of participation in both design and later construction, or an offer to design coupled with an offer of priority (but no contract) in being awarded the tender for work at a later date. The first two of these offers are to consultants, the latter two to designer/sub-contractors. The sorts of design recommendations communicated back from either of these two parties will obviously be affected by the nature of the invitation. One would expect, other things being equal, that the consultant is more likely to communicate a design incorporating his objective professional judgment about the best interests of the client and of the overall design to which he is working. In the second case there is obviously an invitation to communicate a design and specification which will put the designer/sub-contractor in the most favoured position for securing the later tender, or, if he is assured of this already, of carrying it out to his best advantage.

17. For all those involved in this phase of the process, the problem arises of the need for continuous intercommunication between interdependent activities independently carried out. A technical consultant

(or a quantity surveyor) is asked for information or advice concerning the architect's design at some particular point. By the time the consultant has arrived at his answer and communicated this back, the situation described in the original communication may no longer hold. Thus his reply is no longer relevant. With the pressures of time and cost involved it is obviously desirable that all the separate activities necessary for design should go on concurrently, but as they are interdependent how can this be done without the risk of the work of each invalidating the work of others?

18. In exploring this problem we gained the impression that in the early part of this phase formal techniques of communication are not used as fully as they might be. Do the architect and the consultant both insist on a full interchange of information and the development of common understanding in the first exchanges between them? What is, in effect, a full brief could be more fully and usefully used for these communications with the requirements mentioned in paragraph 12. We suspect that a lot of informal traffic occurs at this time with very little formal confirmation. It appears also that more thought and planning with this problem in mind might increase the value of the design meeting as a means of communicating information between the many consultants involved in the common task of the overall design.

19. Paradoxically we also have the impression that the formal communication technique mainly used at later stages of the design phase, the sketch plan, does not ease the problem of constant intercommunication between concurrently developing design activities.* It is limited to two dimensions, is relatively slow to produce and needs interpretation, particularly into the three dimensions which are being planned for. At the present time, because of the nature of sketch plans, we suspect that there is also a good deal of unnecessary information passed in the process of communicating between the designers It occurs to us that an approach to easing this problem could be made from the starting point of an analysis of the way design decisions by any of the parties affect the developing decisions of others. This could form the basis for setting up a system of rapid intercommunication such that relevant information was passed in a simpler, less

---

* For simplicity we are using the term sketch plan to cover all scaled drawings, including sections.

cumbersome and speedier form than the exchange of sketch plans. The use of some coding technique could possibly be of value for achieving this, but detailed research into the operations involved and the interdependence of decision and information would be required as a first step in exploring such a possibility.

20. Obtaining approvals is mentioned under this phase. This is the point in the process at which their effects must be known and taken account of. We are using the term approvals here to cover not only the requirements of the various planning authorities, but also the requirements of bye-laws and of the client. The communications required for obtaining approvals from outside the building team (and we include the client in the team) are largely in prescribed form and, apart from delay, do not of themselves raise serious difficulties as communications. Client approvals will often tend to be dominated by money and/or time required for completion. Client approvals become particularly difficult when the client is the committee of a public body, in this case the design team must at times continue to find a way of satisfying what are often conflicting demands of sections of such a corporate client. When such difficulties arise at this stage however, it can be because communications at the investigation and brief-preparing phase have not been adequately handled, as discussed in paragraph 13. But with a public authority the most settled brief can be upset by changes in other parts of the organisation. A change in financial policy, for example, can interfere with the settled decisions of a housing committee.

21. This raises again the question of optimisation. In the case of design it shows itself as the need to find the best balance between the constraints of the approvals which must be accepted, as well as the need for all parties to the design process to accept some limitation on the best (or optimal) design decision for the part of the whole each is responsible for. The structural engineer, for example, will find that he will not be able to achieve the simplest or optimum design for the structure because it interferes with architectural or other requirements. The same is true of the other consultants and of the architect himself. He too will find that he is unable to design the most elegant building possible because he must meet the requirements of the structural consultant and others. The process of deciding this balance of sub-optimal solutions to all the parts in order to reach the best solution for the whole is another case of optimisation. We sus-

pect that if this process and the particular criteria which determine it were better known to all concurrently designing parts of the same project, much design effort would not be wasted and there would be more useful communication between them - and in many instances less irritation.

Phase 4. Preparing Contract Documents Obtaining Final Approvals

22. "Efficiency in building operations depends on the quality of relationship between the building owner, the professions - architect, surveyor, engineer - and the contractors and sub-contractors"... "There is a good deal of criticism of lack of cohesion between the architect and his professional colleagues and the builder"

Sir Harold Emmerson (18)

23. It is during this phase of the building process that the developing project must quit the shore of the professional area of the industry and make the tricky passage to the other shore of the commercial area. Our experience in the industry is in line with the findings of Sir Harold Emmerson quoted above, with the exception of the role of the quantity surveyor. We see this role, in its traditional form anyway, more as St. Christopher assisting in the passage rather than being firmly planted on either shore. It is the bill of quantities prepared by the quantity surveyor which, again speaking of the traditional model, permits sufficient communication between the two areas to allow the passage of the project from the one area to the other.

24. In addition to the bill of quantities the principal formal communications associated with this phase are drawings (including schedules), specification information, and information about contract conditions.

25. We have already seen enough of this phase of the building process to know that the permutations and combinations of this pattern of communications are very numerous. Contracts can be made on the basis of highly detailed bills, or they can be made without any bills. They can be made with nothing more than the briefest sketch plans or with full sets of working drawings. They can be made without any specifications except those customarily annexed by the quantity surveyor as preambles in the bill, and without any annotations

or they can be made with detailed specifications and full annotations to the bill. The principal determinant of what form the communications shall take in this phase is the prior decision as to the nature of the contract which is to apply. This decision about relationships also has considerable implications for the nature of the communications pattern that shall develop through later phases of the building project.

26. By the nature of the contract we do not simply mean its general type, such as, for example, a package deal, a negotiated contract, a selected tender or an open tender.* We mean something rather more detailed. Under each of these main headings there can be considerable variety. Within a package deal, for example, we know of cases where there was nothing like a bill of quantities at all, and others where there was a full bill. With negotiated contracts the same thing applies. Even contracts decided by competition do not necessarily involve a bill as a basis of competition.

27. However, when cases are looked at in detail one finds that the claim of the bill (and its original justification) to represent and fully describe the structure which will finally emerge is never fully substantiated. At its fullest, in the case of some public authorities who have the reputation for providing 'full documentation', the building implied in the bill is never completely the same as the structure which finally emerges. Client, architect, or "snag" induced variations invariably alter it to some extent. In many cases the building described in the bill and that delineated by the omissions and additions of the final account can be very widely disparate. Indeed, it was not until we concluded that the bill of quantities is usually a hypothe-

---

* An open tender is arrived at as the result of a competition open to all comers. This can allow the contract to go to a lowest bidder with doubtful financial or technical capacity for the job. To avoid this many contracts are offered for competition only among a selected list of builders known to have adequate capacity for the job. A negotiated contract is arrived at without competition by negotiation with one pre-determined builder, usually at an early stage in the building process. In a package deal contract - also called a turn-key contract or all-in service - the client has a single relationship to a main contractor who takes responsibility for all functions, employing or hiring professional help.

tical construct and not necessarily a fully accurate description of reality, despite its detail, that we began to understand the communication processes it serves. Consider in this connection the number of bills which are issued with sections, or are indeed in their entirety marked "Provisional", but which still serve their contractual purposes. Final confirmation of this conclusion is provided by the use of the Master Bill by some of the members of CLASP in their competitions for letting serial tenders.* This bill describes in traditional detail a purely hypothetical building that it is never intended shall exist.

28. That the bill of quantities in its traditional form has little function beyond its contractual purpose seems to be accepted by most parties. This we have heard from builders:

> ".....we must admit that the Standard Method of Measurement is not very much use to a builder when it comes to planning his operations on the site."

> "Some different presentation of information to the builder could help materially in enabling us to plan our work."

29. Many quantity surveyors are of the same opinion. For example:

> "We know it (the bill) is essentially a tendering document and it is not very much use to a contractor for the things he has to do for planning his contract, controlling his costs, and so on."

30. This is not to say that the bill of quantities does not usually fulfil its primary contractual purpose of providing a uniform basis for making lump sum offers and schedules of rates for pricing variations. Our impression is, however, that if the true nature of the bill as a hypothetical construct were more widely understood, less tedious, more economical and equally effective techniques could be found for achieving these same ends. Moreover, such redesigned techniques could be set up with the needs of construction planning and control in

---

* CLASP is a group, mainly of local authorities, who have combined to exploit the advantages of standardised modular design and large scale factory pre-fabrication. The serial contract is a contract for the erection of several buildings, all using the CLASP system, which are contemplated but the designs for which are not yet finalised.

mind so that analyses done for 'contract documentation' would be of much greater direct and immediate use to the construction phase. Work being done on elemental and operational bills are currently developing moves in this direction.

31. Given the different size of buildings, and particularly the time pressures, of modern conditions compared with those prevailing at the time the bill of quantities technique for arriving at a contract arose, the persistence of the traditional procedures can lead to serious tangles in communications. By traditional practice the bill, as a representation of the building actually to be produced, was taken off from the working drawings which were to be the detailed instructions to the builder. Nowadays they almost always have to be worked up from a lot less information than this. This means that if the quantity surveyor is to produce anything like a complete bill he must initiate a considerable volume of communications to the architect to get his decisions about many details which are not settled at this stage, and often for good reasons cannot be. This situation is not new, nor is the architect as the scapegoat for it, as is shown by the following report from an RICS discussion in 1901:

> "It was quite impossible for the surveyor to take out quantities from drawings such as sometimes come from the architect's office, imperfectly finished and possibly incorrect" (8, p. 254)

32. But then, as now, quantity surveyors were concerned with this problem and were suggesting ways round it. The following is a report of the contribution of a quantity surveyor to the same discussion:*

> "He saw no object in making the quantities part of the contract. They were only a means of obtaining and fixing the price and were not part and parcel of the drawings and specifications from which the job should be carried out, although he thought it wise to deposit them as priced bills for any variations ..."
>
> (ibid. p. 244)

33. Although bills of quantities have long since become part of the

---

* This quotation refers to the time before quantities became part of the RIBA Form of Contract, when specifications were still prepared by architects and were contract documents. For many years now contractors have refused in most cases to make lump sum bids without bills

normal contract (and the specification has ceased to be a contract document), techniques allowing contracts to be made without detailed bills of quantities, even on a competitive basis, have existed concurrently and quantity surveyors are now developing them further (12). These techniques can still involve bills of quantities in the post-contract stages, but as means of providing realistic descriptions of buildings, with considerably enhanced value for the builder, as distinct from hypothetical constructs for settling schedules of rates. This use of the bill as a technique of materials accountancy will obviously have implications for its own development. One would expect it will become less tied to the Standard Method and the traditional trade divisions, and take more account of the needs of modern construction control.

34. It is claimed against contract procedures which do not use bills of quantities that they cost the client more. About this we do not know, and we suspect that nobody else has any reliable evidence. The counter-claim is that if the cost of having a building earlier could be known, which these procedures allow, and as far as we know this exercise has never been undertaken either, there might indeed be a long term saving to the client, even if immediately he pays more.

35. The complaint of lack of design information at contract stage is a hardy perennial in the building process. Even the firm price contract which, following its lapse during the war, has become more popular in recent years, particularly with the Government, has not been able to overcome this difficulty, although the provision of 'full documentation' at the time of contract is a condition for the operation of the system. It has recently been reported in a survey in one region of the country that only 25 per cent. of firm price contracts were completed with what was described as adequate documentation (42).

36. This raises the question of what is adequate documentation at this phase of the building process. We find ourselves unable to answer this question and we would suggest that, at the present stage of objective knowledge about the part played by information at various points in the building process, this question cannot be answered, only hypothesised about. What is adequate information for any kind of contractual arrangement apart from the empirical definition of "that amount which allows a contract to be made"? Further, what is the adequate amount of information that the contractor needs at

contract stage to allow him to undertake construction planning? Our impression is that what this is claimed to be is often a lot more than is really required. Experience of other arrangements than the traditional contract, package deals and negotiated contracts for example, show that not only planning but work on the site can be undertaken before many quite important design decisions have been made.

37. We have found practice in respect to specifications and schedules very various. At some point in the building process the quality of materials, finishes and design details must be decided. There is considerable lack of consistency or even information, not only about when these decisions are taken but about who takes them. Some architects have been described to us as 'fussy' because they insist on taking all these decisions themselves. Others are content to let the quantity surveyor, the contractor or even the workman on the job effectively decide many of these matters.

38. The request for the annotation of bills we find more difficult to deal with.* If, as we suspect - and the quotations from builders above also support this - the bill is usually used only as a tender document, we cannot see that relating it closely to the usually preliminary drawings from which the bill has been prepared serves much useful purpose. Here again, more actual information about the use bills and other tender documents have, or could have, in the construction phase is required.

Phase 5. Preparing and Agreeing Contract
Setting up Construction Team

39. Working up and agreeing the contract is much more a routine process than it is a phase requiring the making of design and technical communications. By working up the contract we are referring to the process of making communications to tenderers by the client or his professional advisers, getting replies and taking a decision. It covers the formalised routines involved in letting, receiving and deciding tenders. In the course of this process technical and design information may be communicated between the parties but this is usually to

---

* Annotated bills have a reference against each item indicating its location in the building, as shown on the drawings from which the bills were prepared.

elucidate other points at issue than strictly design or technical matters. The communications in this phase tend to have to do with settling relative positions of financial interest and contractual conditions and can involve communications with others than the parties normally associated with the building process, for example, lawyers and insurance companies.

40. Just what communications are required and how they are developed again depends very much on the nature of the contract which is being entered into. The formalisation of a package deal contract is obviously a different sort of process from that involved in an open tender, a selected tender, a negotiated tender, the type of competitive but "unmeasured" tender mentioned previously, or a serial tender.

41. The outcome of this procedure is usually some form of legally binding document but the complication it involves can be gauged from the time taken for the principal parties in the building industry to agree on the revision of the forms for this function which have recently been published under the sponsorship of the RIBA, and which some claim are already obsolescent.

42. As far as we know there is no comprehensive information on the range in the variety of types of contractual arrangements in the building industry,* nor any knowledge of the implications of the different types for later phases of the building process and the different patterns of communication they generate.

43. In addition to the legally binding activities involved in the working up and agreeing of the contract, there is an area which has a lot of traditional ritual surrounding it. The procedures, particularly of some public bodies, for calling for tenders, for opening them, and for passing information to tenderers, is subject to a good deal of custom, which although having historical justification now has little sanction other than tradition and goodwill. A builder discovered in taking a cover price,**

---

* We understand the Q.S. Committee of the RICS is currently making such a census.

** A builder "takes a cover" if he does not want to accept an invitation to tender for a job, but deems it impolitic to refuse outright. He will ask another builder whom he finds out is tendering seriously for the job to give him a price to put in which is high enough to avoid his making the lowest or near lowest offer.

for example, although not behaving illegally, is considered to have broken the rules. In the same way a client or a client's agent who, for no good reason, opens more than one priced bill is similarly considered to be caught off side. And to open all the bills is to ask for boycott.

44. The setting up of the construction team is mainly the responsibility of the main contractor. Once he has been awarded the contract, he takes on the role of sponsor of the construction team. In this role he must build up and maintain the appropriate pattern of relationships to control the interdependent activities whose joint contributions will emerge as the finished building.

45. The communications involved in this process are obviously very various. There are many formal communications which may include legal agreements of various kinds. There are also many informal communications of a variety of kinds, including the Dutch auction, as a method of choosing sub-contractors. We understand that this latter procedure is initiated as often by the sub-contractors as it is by the main contractor. It would certainly seem that such factors as personal acquaintance, goodwill or favours owed often come into play in the setting up of the construction team.

46. The main contractor, in undertaking the sponsorship of the construction team, has the function of optimising the mix of resources and skills called for. This would appear to be a technically simpler exercise in optimisation than in the design phase, as it is guided by the simpler and technically more easily handled single criterion of maximising a profitable financial return. To ensure that the optimum pattern he has decided on is realised, the main contractor needs to maintain a series of communications through the construction process. This pattern of communications on the site is essentially two way. In one direction it is a monitoring function of gathering information, covering not only the on-going work but also the cues for the co-ordination of future work, the arrival of supplies, labour and plant, ordering ahead, etc. The main contractor is in most cases equally concerned with ensuring the early departure from the site of plant or equipment for which is paying an expensive hire. All these functions require the constant flow of information to a co-ordinating point allowing decisions to be taken. These in turn lead to a flow of information outwards to a multiplicity of

others who must take subsequent action if the whole process is to proceed as planned.

47. Many of these communications are informal, on the telephone or orally. Just what the nature of this overall pattern is is not known in comprehensive detail as distinct from partial records. We would suggest that a complete and detailed study of the whole pattern of communications on and relating to the operations on building sites would well repay study.

48. A high point of construction team communication is of course the site meeting. This too is an institution that might well be considerably improved as a technique of communication if its various interlocking functions were thoroughly understood. As well as supplying the need for technical co-ordination the site meeting also usually has a function, in terms of developing and maintaining relationships, of relative influence and control among all concerned. Of particular interest is the relationship of others than those directly involved in the construction team to site meetings of different kinds, in particular the relationship of the architect and the consultants.

49. The nature of the relationships between the parties again will have a big influence on the pattern of communications generated in and around the construction team. If the builder is nominated early in the building process it is possible for him both to receive and make communications relative to the processes that precede the setting up of the construction team, but which will affect its working. In such cases the process of setting up the team is slower as it can start much earlier, and it can be relatively complete by the time construction is ready to begin. One of the problems this procedure is said to overcome centres on the relationship between main contractors and nominated sub-contractors which can be a source of many difficulties (33). If the main contractor is himself nominated early in the building process he can be a party to the nomination of sub-contractors. Whether this procedure with its claimed advantages is, in fact, often realised we are not in a position to know with assurance. We have had reports from builders who have experience of early nomination that range from a close contact between the builder and the designers to a situation not essentially different from that prevailing under the more traditional type of entry for the builder. Some builders have said they prefer not to be involved in the design phase and do not see any great

advantage, either for themselves or for the building process as a whole, of their being so included.

Phase 6. Construction to Completion

50. This phase of the process is a continuation of the latter part of the previous phase, and much of what has been said there applies through construction to completion.

51. Apart from the points already made about the communications required for the control of the construction team, as the job develops there is the question of communications off the site to do with directions for the process itself. In this respect there can be some complication of roles. A sub-contractor who has also designed the work, for example, will need to communicate instructions to the main contractor in his role as designer, but be under the control of the main contractor in his function as a sub-contractor. It is often reported that this position causes difficulties in communications during the construction phase. Such a sub-contractor, it is said, feels he has a special relationship to the members of the design team with whom he claims a right of communication, particularly to the architect, irrespective of the intervening role of the builder. Exactly what effect this has on communications, and in turn on the effectiveness of the building process, has not been studied in detail, but would obviously be worth such attention.

52. At this time the builder can suffer from the confusion in communications that has been generated in earlier stages of the building process, particularly those mentioned under Phase 4 above. Here we quote from two quantity surveyors:-

> "There is a practice whereby the negatives (of drawing prints) are altered during the work of the quantity surveyor so that there is absolutely no record at all of what they were like originally. They are sometimes altered without the quantity surveyor even knowing that they have been altered, so that neither side knows where the dickens they are by the time it comes to contract."

> "It would be very nice if it could get to the stage where the architect altered his negative to suit what we have taken off. The trouble is, in my experience, between the time the contract has been tendered for and the working drawings have

been got out the negative is again altered. Nobody knows what is going on. The result is that we get the builder saying "Something here does not match up." There is no variation order, it is just a different drawing altogether. It bears the same number and date and there are no other amendments added to it."

A comment from a builder:-

"I do find quite frequently when I go on to a site that the poor wretched foreman, who has no access to contract drawings and things that may be filed away in a safe, is just building from the wrong drawings. How is he to know? He has bills of quantities on his desk and I do not think it is asking too much to put down a list of the drawings from which those quantities were prepared."

This, however, is not a situation which builders find universally disadvantageous.

"I for one would not be at all put out if I found my foreman working to a set of drawings totally different from the contract drawings. I would start sharpening my pencil and think up all the extras I could claim as a consequence. It is on these items that we make our money."

53. This would appear to arise from a confusion of objectives in communications. One set of drawings is used as a basis for preparing bills of quantities and making a contract. These are not necessarily, or indeed on some occasions advisably, to be taken as working drawings for construction. The prudent builder will insist on another communication for his construction decisions to that which he has had for contract decision.

54. The nature of the relationships existing is obviously crucial in this matter. In the last quotation above it can be seen that a vested interest can exist in faulty communications. Within a package deal arrangement on the other hand the man in charge of construction would have no such vested interest in poor communications from his design colleagues.

55. Indeed the way communications are handled by one construction organisation that we have met depends upon what sort of contract they are working under. If they are working within a competitive contract

all incoming communications are registered and are immediately checked by an estimator and draughtsman who search for any omissions, confusions, or conflicts with previous communications. These are all noted and communicated to the source of the incoming material. It was explained that this is not necessarily to ensure that the difficulties are put straight, they say they can always sort those out themselves, and indeed prefer to, but to cover themselves when it comes to the final account. When this same organisation undertakes a negotiated contract or a package deal the communication channels are much simpler and they insist on keeping them uncluttered with such secondary communications as registration and cross checking. If difficulties arise they are taken up by informal means and quickly rectified.

56. The same sort of thing applies to variation orders and the quantity surveyor's activities in measuring for certification. Within the traditional contract relationship variation orders are communications that almost invariably lead to difficulties for somebody. Where the relationship between the parties is of a different nature the variation order is a communication with much less disturbing implications.

Phase 7. Handing Over and Settling Final Account

57. The communications arising from the inspection by the client's professional advisers on completion are obviously contractual, although they may deal with technical matters. They have to do essentially with the finalisation of the bargaining process involved in buying and selling. They may be informal or they may be quite formal and indeed legal.

58. It is at this time that the bill of quantities, if there is one, is used as an instrument by both parties to get the best deal possible in sorting out variations, which can be extensive and determine financial margins crucial for several parties. We know that under any contractual arrangement differences between the contract price and final account can arise, and for a variety of reasons. We have a strong impression, however, that much of the often prolonged and acrimonious argument associated with settling building accounts, which seldom lead to any party's great advantage but which bring considerable discredit to the industry in the eyes of the public, is avoidable. The discussion under Phase 4 above suggests that the forms of communication commonly employed in making the original

contract are incapable, under modern conditions, despite their impressive bulk, of presenting enough of the relevant information sufficiently accurately for a simple and equitable bargain to be made.

59. The difficulties arising in this phase would seem to be largely due to the accumulation of the results of inadequate communication throughout the whole building process right from its inception. A detailed study of this phenomenon of accumulation, together with the conditions which lead up to it, should do a lot towards improvement, not only for this phase but also for the earlier phases that generate the residues for this final sorting out.

Summing Up

60. Our review of communications in this section leads us to two general conclusions. First, that the main factor lying behind communications difficulties is the nature of the relationships between the communicators. Second, that any attempt at improvement, however limited, cannot hope to achieve any significant degree of success in the absence of much more information than is at present available, about just what job any communication is supposed to do.

61. Over the years various attempts have been made to improve relationships and communications in the industry (14, 69, 43, 34, 41, 33, 18). All have been useful, but none has produced more than minor advances. We suggest that it is the absence of the conditions implied in our two conclusions above that has prevented greater success for these efforts. They have not been able to do more than canvass best opinion and agree general precepts on that basis. The question of relationships is taken up in the next section. The need for information, we hope, has been fully demonstrated in this section.

62. As a beginning we suggest the following as fact-finding tasks, the results of which are prerequisites to the development of better communication techniques and procedures.

> Most clients are very ill-informed of the services the industry can offer. As a result many clients never achieve adequate satisfaction to their building needs. All the members of the public are not equally likely to become clients. How can those interested in building (including planners) identify the groups most likely to do so, and anticipate their needs with appropriate information?

What are the usual types of problems faced by the client and his advisers in the very important tasks of investigation and arriving at a brief? What techniques are known within the industry and in other fields that could help with these problems?

Just how is the design team usually built up, and what is the nature of its relationships and communications techniques in terms of helping or hindering the common task of creating a total design?

How many different kinds of contract actually exist? On what information are they settled? What, in fact, are the minimum amounts of information required for contracts of different kinds to be satisfactorily made?

What are the actual timings, contents and techniques of the communications now going to the construction team? What, in these respects, is the objectively-determined minimum to ensure effectiveness in different circumstances?

What is the nature of communications within the construction team? What, again on an objectively-determined basis, are the communication needs of efficient construction control?

SECTION III

A CONSIDERATION OF FACTORS AFFECTING ROLES AND RELATIONSHIPS IN THE BUILDING TEAM

1. The consideration of the techniques and uses of communications discussed in the last section makes it clear that the way communications are used, and indeed what communications are used, depends very much on the pattern of roles involved and the relationships existing between them.

2. This was a general impression we had very early in our contact with the building industry. One of our difficulties in the fieldwork was to get people to discuss techniques of communication with us. Such discussion almost invariably led straight into considerations of the divisions of responsibility and of relationships in the building team. Our conclusion in this respect agrees with that of the great majority of people in the industry with whom we discussed this question. Namely, that the pattern of relationships and the divisions of responsibility in any building team have much more effect on the way communications function than have any particular aspects of the techniques of communication themselves. This of course is not to say that the techniques could not be improved, but such improvement would appear to be a marginal contribution to improving co-ordination and cohesion in the building team. Indeed, before we learnt this lesson we were several times accused of being naive if, as it appeared, we expected to be able to recommend anything leading to significant change merely through the improvement of the techniques of communication. We were several times told that if people's relationships with those carrying other parts of the job could be improved the question of communications would very soon take care of itself. To this we would only add - if the information needed to develop improved techniques is available.

3. This section then is the result of the study of the patterns of the division of responsibilities and of relationships in the building team to which we were thus led. We are not attempting to set up a comprehensive typology to embrace all the types of patterns that exist. This was a task we very early realised was much too involved and complex for us, with the time and resources at our disposal, to take any further than it has already been taken by others (13, 66). We do not think this

task can move forward without fairly large scale survey techniques and some quantification. The field is too complex. Our approach therefore is more in terms of the forces acting on and within the building industry in the past and at the present time that have produced the patterns of relationship and the divisions of function that now exist and which have relevance to the problems of communication. This has led us to make a brief excursion into the history of the industry as well as to get as full an understanding as we can of the nature of the forces which are currently operating to determine the nature of changes presently at work and those likely to develop in the future. We obviously cannot claim to have made a full and comprehensive analysis of these forces. We hope however that we will be able to say enough to allow the next steps in this area to be decided.

Historical Background up to the Eighteenth Century

4. The building industry had a guild type of structure through the Middle Ages and right into the seventeenth century. It was the fire of London in the middle of that century that occasioned the first big change in the structure of the industry. The enormous amount of rebuilding required in London at that time, and the need for this reconstruction to proceed rapidly, was too great a demand on the guild system for it to meet at all adequately. As with many other aspects of English national life, what happens in London becomes the national pattern sooner or later. This challenge was met by a development which was itself in line with the developing bourgeois economic culture of the time, the building craftsman as entrepreneur. The approach of these new men was more concerned with getting the job done and realising on an investment of capital or labour in the quickest and most profitable way than it was concerned with the workmanship or the "delight" of the result. This new approach had obvious advantages in the situation of crisis which the rebuilding of London created.

5. The development of this new organisational technique had of course to start from the pattern existing at that time. Thus the new commercial building units tended to centre round an enterprising master craftsman from one of the old Guilds.* Small enterprises undertaking brick-

---

* There were twelve mediaeval Guilds involved in building. These were: bricklayer/tyler, carpenter, glazier, ironmonger, joiner, mason, painter/stainer, pavier, pewterer, plaisterer, plumber, turner

laying, carpentry, plumbing, etc. sprang up, each controlled by a man from the appropriate Guild background.

6. In order to co-ordinate these economically separated and competing units, working at a rather higher register than previously, some form of co-ordination was required. Under the Guild system with its slower tempo the design function was barely separated from the construction function. The master artisans worked it out among themselves and with the client as they went along. This demand for co-ordination and design were the factors determining the rise of the role of the architect as we know it today. As most of the landlords in London were of the nobility, the architects who were to act on their behalf, were drawn from the ranks of educated gentlemen rather than from the artisan classes. Hence the liberal arts tradition with its broad social perspective still associated with the profession.

7. By the eighteenth century a new pattern had settled for the carrying out of building operations. This is illustrated in Figure III.1. There it can be seen that the architect operates directly for the client and employs the various separate single trade commercial units.

8. An early difficulty that arose with this system was the problem of agreeing the piece-rate price that was the basis of payment. Because they felt at a disadvantage vis-a-vis the architect with his greater education, the groups of artisans would employ a man who was as skilled in calculating as the architect to measure the work they had done and negotiate with the architect for payment on their behalf. These men became known as measurers and operated the system of 'Measure and Value". As measurers became more skilled at pressing the claims of the craftsmen, so, in self defence, the architect would also employ a measurer to act on his behalf. This situation gave rise to intense and bitter complaints and litigation at the expense of the public and to the detriment of the quality and efficiency of building.

The First Half of the Nineteenth Century

9. Towards the end of the eighteenth century the pattern of the building process, set out in Figure III.1. began to prove

FIG. III 1

18th CENTURY

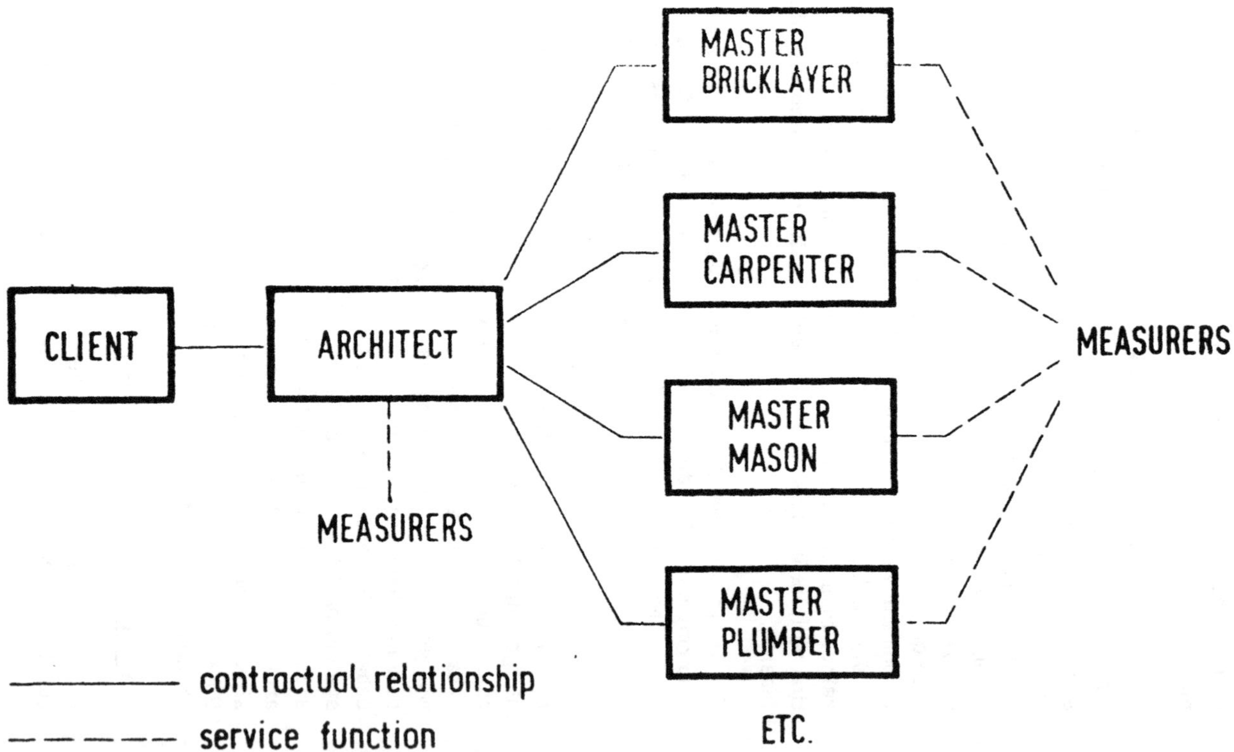

unsatisfactory. The industrial revolution was making increasing demands for domestic and public as well as industrial building. At the end of the century and into the nineteenth century the country also suffered the stresses and demands of warfare. The existing method of organising the building process was no longer adequate to the demands made upon it. It was cumbersome, uneconomic and inefficient and, in effect, society would not put up with it any longer. During the Napoleonic Wars the Government stepped in and in order to encourage economy and despatch in building it passed a regulation that each job had to be under the control of one responsible contractor. This made mandatory a system that had already begun to develop.

10. This system developed by one of the craftsman entrepreneurs taking charge of the whole construction process through a single contract from the architect. This enterprising craftsman was usually a bricklayer. In an age when brick was the principal building material, it was the bricklayer more than any other craftsman who had the greatest familiarity with the building as a whole. Also, as the foundations were built in brick, he was the man who was responsible for making these and undertaking the excavation. Thus, technically, he was the man most suited to become the general contractor. Being a tradesman in a rather larger way than the others, the bricklayer also tended to have more capital at his disposal.

11. The main contractor very quickly incorporated the other trades within his own organisation, though of course this process was not complete in all cases. There was still some contracting by separate trades, but it was now the main contractor, not the architect, who let what now became "sub" contracts to other trades. This pattern is set out in Figure III. 2. For simplicity, the contractual relationship, legally to the client, is shown on the diagrams as with his agent the architect.

12. It will be seen that the measurer has given way to the quantity surveyor. This development did not become fully established until nearly the middle of the nineteenth century. The Royal Exchange, built in 1842, is said to be the first major building project on which a bill of quantities in anything like its modern form was first used.

13. The development of quantity surveying was as a response to the need to find a common basis for comparing the bids of main contractors for a job. Each would guess at the requirements of the drawings differently. To meet this need there were developments by various more enterprising measurers in the technique of measurement from drawings. The result was the bill of quantities and the emergence of the role of the quantity surveyor.

14. In the early days the bill of quantities was thought of as a service to the builder to allow him to arrive at his contract figure. He was thus employed and paid by the builder. It was common practice right into the twentieth century for the architect also to employ a quantity surveyor in parallel with the man employed by the builder. The practice of the builder paying the quantity surveyor, even when only one was used by joint agreement, persisted into the present century and was still extant at the time of the Simon report in 1944.

15. The development of main contracting from an earlier system of divided trades, and its incorporation of these trades within itself, gave the form to the bill of quantities that it has today. It is broken down by the (originally Mediaeval) trade headings that the early main contractors would use as their divisions in costing. From their days of earlier separation the different trades had developed their own particular techniques for the Measure and Value method and these naturally went forward to be incorporated in the quantity surveyors' techniques for working up the bill.

Late Nineteenth Century and to the Present

16. The pattern set out in Figure III. 2 did not persist very long. The reason for this was the rapid development of technology in building that came with the increased pace of industrial development through the nineteenth century. The first major event in this respect was probably the invention of Portland cement in 1825. It was of course some time before it became a standard material, and in its early days, as might be expected, where it was used it was handled by a specialist sub-contractor. When it became a sufficiently standard technique, being on the "heavy" side, it became incorporated into the sphere of the main contractor.

17. About the middle of the century the tempo of technological change increased. Steel, or in its early days wrought iron, was one of the

FIG. III 2.

1st HALF OF 19th CENTURY

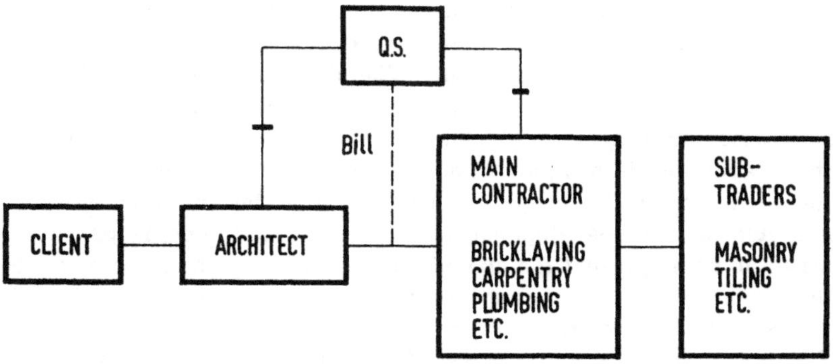

—+— Only one of these relationships exists at one time for the same job

FIG. III 3.

LATE 19th CENTURY & TO PRESENT DAY

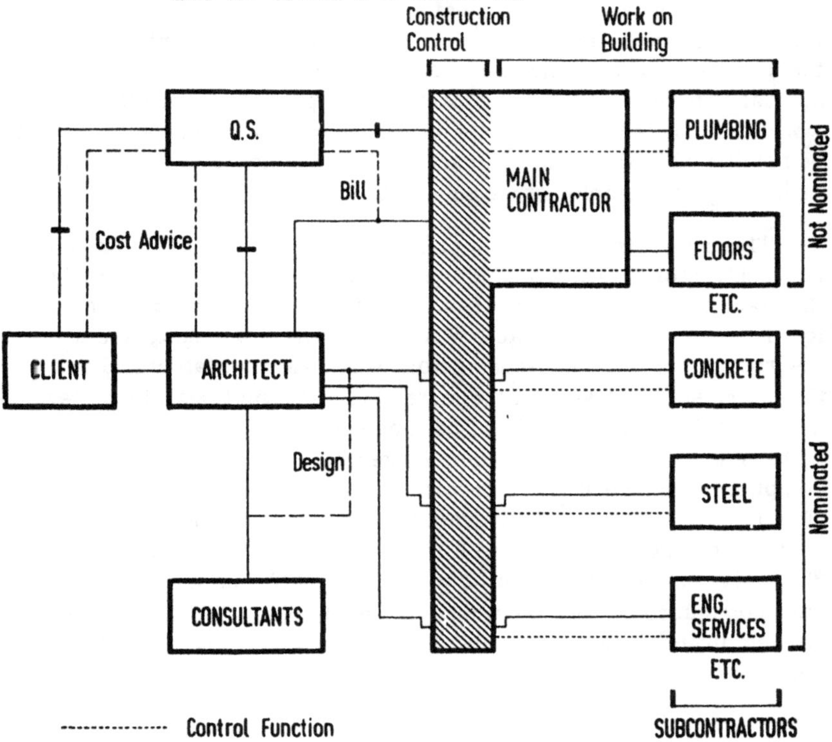

-------------- Control Function

first of the new materials to come into building. Later, ornamental brickwork, terra-cotta and other specialist materials became incorporated. In all cases the new materials and, in due course, the new techniques arriving with electrical and mechanical engineering (central heating, lifts, etc.) came into the industry through sub-contracting by specialists in handling them. The skills of these specialists were obviously needed in those aspects of the design that involved their particular material or technique. They thus became involved with the architect in design. In due course specialist designing became separated out from specialist sub-contracting in the role of the consultant, but this development did not eliminate the designer/sub-contractor role. In that the specialist designer, in either role, could be held responsible for part of the overall design, the relationship of responsibility between these roles and that of the architect as responsible for the whole became somewhat confused. By the turn of the last century, the picture showed very much the pattern set out in Figure III. 3.

18. A new development in the structure of the industry shown in this diagram is the use of the nominated sub-contractor. This development was begun by more enterprising architects who wanted to use the new techniques or materials and who would apply to the appropriate specialist to help with those aspects of design. To ensure that the work was carried out correctly this specialist sub-contractor would be nominated in the main contract. The main contractor would also, as before, still employ other sub-contractors directly.

19. The increasing proportion of building work being undertaken by sub-contractors meant that the proportional amount done directly by the main contractor became less. He was still however responsible for the erection of the whole building. He was expected to see that the work done by the sub-contractors was done adequately and that they were supplied with all the materials and conditions which they needed to do their work. This became known as "attendance". As building construction has become larger in scale and technically more complex, so attendance has become a much more complex function. This is the section on the diagram labelled 'construction control'. Indeed, in modern conditions with the main contractor often undertaking 30 per cent or less of the building work himself - in our field work we have come across one case where the main contractor in fact is doing nothing directly - the provision of this control becomes the principal function of the main contractor.

20. The quantity surveyors continued to develop their techniques of measurement, although it took them a long time to standardise their methods of doing this. It was not until 1922 that the first agreed handbook on a method of measurement was produced.

21. The effects of the expansion of industry and population growth on the price of urban land, the development of new but more costly building materials and techniques, and the growth in the size of buildings all tended to force up both the unit and overall cost of building. In these circumstances the discrepancies between estimated and contract prices and final account became much more significant and led to increasing client dissatisfaction.

22. The quantity surveyor with his techniques of analysing jobs for estimating purposes was the obvious best equipped member of the building team to assist with this problem. For many years quantity surveyors had made a practice of collating information from past jobs as a basis for providing advice to architects and clients about the estimated expenditure required for buildings that were being contemplated or designed. Initially these techniques were very much rule of thumb. As time went on methods of collating a wider range of data and more accurate techniques of analysis were developed, until the position has been reached during the years since the last war when the quantity surveyor is able to provide a service of high accuracy to clients and architects. Cost planning is the best known of these techniques. We therefore refer to this emerging role in the field of quantity surveying as that of the cost planner.*

23. This is a very significant development for quantity surveying as, for the first time, it gives to the quantity surveyor a claim to full professional status. The traditional function of the quantity surveyor of measuring, either from drawings for the bill of quantities or 'as made' for certification and final account, was less than a full professional function. He drew the chess board and made the pieces and even kept the score, as it were, but was not involved in the game. A full professional role requires not only an expertise in a particular field but the participation through the acceptance of expert judgment directly in any decision-making process. The bill of quantities and 'as made' measurements, although a necessary piece of equipment for

* Cost planning is also known as expenditure planning or budgetary control.

decisions, do not directly affect them as does the judgment or advice of the architect or consultant, for example. With the development of the cost planner role, however, the judgment and advice as well as the expertise of a quantity surveyor is brought to bear in the decision-making of the building process. What he has to say will directly affect design or contractual decisions, and what is more he will be held responsible for the outcome. He is now in a role of high discretion. The role of the quantity surveyor as measurer is a role of very low discretion, being fully prescribed by the procedures laid down in the Method of Measurement and the routines of taking off, abstracting and working up. In theory this could be (and we believe in some cases is) fully prescribed as the programme for a machine operation. The discretion called for by professional judgement cannot be mechanised. It is into the design function that this new cost estimating function of the quantity surveyor fits. Originally it was as a service to the architect who had to advise the client about cost estimates, and also to guide him in design decisions. More recently quantity surveyors have been making a direct relationship with the client for estimating purposes.

24. A much more recent development is that of cost control by the quantity surveyor, drawing on the same techniques and sources of information as for cost planning. The functions of this developing service have been described (in part) by the Cost Research Panel of the Quantity Surveyors' Committee of the RICS as the quantity surveyor's ability to "advise on economies that might be embodied in the design, such as the design of shuttering in relation to repetitive structual components, and the use of prefabricated and precast techniques etc., and to advise on the boundary of responsibility between the main and sub-contractors' (56, p. 149). If the quantity surveyor can develop cost control as a service to these functions, he will obviously participate fundamentally in the decisions of construction control, and so add another fully professional function to his role, this time in the construction area of the industry.

25. These developments in the role of the quantity surveyor, although having promising but not yet fully tested value for the building process particularly in their contribution to co-ordination for the design phase, the construction phase and overall, cut right to the heart of the "demarcation" problems of the building team. If the claims made for them are pressed too extravagantly or too hastily, or if

resistance to them is too defensively irrational, they could create more trouble in building team relationships than they could contribute value to the building process (16).

26. We have not been able to discover when the negotiated contract first emerged in the building industry. It seems clear, however, that it is forces affecting the industry internally and externally since the last war that have caused its recent considerable development to the point where it is now one of the well accepted bases of the relationships in the building team.

27. The pressure for reconstruction after the blitz, the backlog of building which had built up over the war and the building needs of the full economy that developed in the forties and early fifties put tremendous pressure on the building industry. Associated with this situation there was a resurgence of purely commercial building activity by developers. Post-war city building has also tended to be on a larger scale than previously. They were, too, the various town and country planning regulations introduced after the war that added to the confusions and delays of the building process. In these conditions the delay and the cost of following the traditional method of competitive tender, with its long period of preparation to the point of settling the contract and getting site work started, was a cause of increasing irritation, particularly to clients. The reduction of costs and time that the negotiated contract promised gave this form of contractual relationship a good deal of popularity as a result. Members of the building team were also dissatisfied with the working of the traditional procedure and were happy to accept the change. This was particularly true of main contractors who had a proprietary system, usually prefabricated, or specialised equipment which they were eager to use. The negotiated contract allowed the main contractor to participate in the design process so that he had a much better chance of ensuring that his system or equipment was used and, where it was, that its advantages were fully exploited in the design.

28. The negotiated contract for the first time allows a relationship across the contractual area between the professional and commercial sides of the industry. It entails both immediate and longer term implications for change from the traditional in the patterns of relationship and responsibility for all the roles involved. It is such apparently small innovations, introduced to help with currently felt difficulties, that provide the growing points for the future. As the industry learns

to work with and adjust them, so it evolves re-definitions of its roles better adapted to meet the changed demands it must face.

29. The points made so far in this section, concerning the relationship between the forces outside and inside the industry and their effects upon the existing roles and relationships in the building team, are summarised in the attached table, at the end of this section.

30. It will be noticed that the supply side of the industry is not included in these considerations. This is not because we do not consider manufacturers, suppliers and builders merchants as unimportant in their contribution to the building process. Our subject of attention is communications, and in this respect our brief study of the industry has not thrown up communications problems of central importance between these and other members of the building team. Indeed, their communications with builders, their usual contacts in the building team, seem to be good (51). In as much as their communications with architects are not, the plans of the National Council of Building Material Producers for a technical catalogue designed mainly for architects promises to remedy this.

The Contemporary Situation

31. In the attached table the pattern of relationships and divisions of responsibility that represents the most developed consolidated position in these respects is shown as position A. Beyond that some examples are given of emerging models in the building industry today. This presentation is, of course, for exemplification only; it makes no claims to being exhaustive.

32. The development in other industries of diversifying fabrication and distinguishing it from assembly, particularly in the motor industry and the consumer durable industries, has provided models for similar thinking and developments in building. For several decades there have been efforts to develop standardisation of components and prefabrication in building. More recently modular systems to rationalise these processes have been developing. For the building industry the separation of fabrication from assembly has additional merits of allowing much of the work to be taken off the site and into the more advantageous conditions of the factory.

33. A condition that was necessary for this development in other industries was a large market allowing for the high level of production

without which these procedures have no advantage. A difficulty with the traditional approach to building is the lack of such a large long-term programme of production. In the years since the war it has been obvious to several internal sponsors of local authorities that between them their clients' organisations could ensure such a programme. The result has been the development of client/design team consortia, such as CLASP, SCOLA and 5M. These consortia extend responsibility right across the design and contractual areas of the process, but construction, although largely determined by what has gone before, is an activity which remains, in most cases, outside the consortium. To ensure that the advantages of long-term stable programmes should be realised on the construction side also, the serial contract was developed.

34. With the increasing confusion of responsibilities and instability of pattern in the structure of the building team, clients, particularly sophisticated clients, have in recent years become increasingly dissatisfied in their dealings with the industry. It occurred to such people that, if the whole building process could be brought together under a single control which was directly responsible to themselves, a greater effectiveness might be achieved. The way this was done in some cases was to develop further the already existing procedure of the client taking charge himself and undertaking direct labour building.

35. At the same time many contractors were dissatisfied with the low margins that they were getting in their enterprises. They believed that this was largely generated during the processes of design and by the traditional forms of contract that were largely outside their control. These men had a common interest with dissatisfied clients in wanting to establish single co-ordination over the whole building project. This led to the emergence of the package deal.

36. It should be reported that all builders are by no means convinced that the package deal is the answer to their problems.

> "The Architect saying you must, the Q.S. saying you can't afford to, the planning boys saying they won't let you, the Arty-Tarty Commission saying you shouldn't, and half of Victoria Street stirring the pot - I don't want any of that malarkey! When they've made up their minds what they want, let them come to me with something I can put a price to and get on and build - and keep out

of my hair while I build it! The package deal? A package of trouble for the builder! Whoever made any money out of that malarkey stuff? By the time you've paid for the carpets and the pot plants and the pink gins, you're out of pocket."

37. The experience of clients in undertaking direct labour building has not by any means been invariably happy (26). Many such clients began to doubt whether they were really qualified to control such a large undertaking in an area which was beyond their usual competence. At the same time many sophisticated clients who wished to see some overall control of the process established were not happy to achieve this by putting themselves entirely into the hands of the main contractor in his role as package dealer. From this situation there has emerged the role of professional contractor. As far as we know this has not manifested itself in this country, but it does exist in New York, and under present day conditions this can mean that it could easily appear in this country quite soon. This is particularly so as the instance that we know of in New York is the new building recently built over Grand Central Station, for which a British developer is part client. The complete control of the construction side of this project was being undertaken on a professional fee-paying basis by an organisation which takes full responsibility for sponsoring the building team and for all its operations throughout the construction phase. It has no building operatives in its direct employment, only a small staff of labour for "general housekeeping". This development cuts right across the traditional relationships between professionalism and design on the one side, and commercialism and construction on the other.

38. Finally, something of the current situation in respect to the external forces affecting the industry should be mentioned. In the eyes of society at large, the present perception of the industry is not good. All the more serious daily and weekly papers have within recent months given attention to what is considered to be the ill-health of the building industry, its low productivity, and particularly the assumed poor return it is giving for the very large share of the industry's income that society as a whole pays for directly.

39. There are, too, the implications for several building team roles of the continuing trend to industrialisation and prefabrication, not merely of components but of whole sections of a building. What effect

will this sort of development have on the traditional responsibilities of the architect and the builder, for example? Another source of pressure, which may have quite important effects, is the demand that will be put on the industry if the NEDC's planned rate of growth for the economy is realised over future years.

40. The Government has also shown some concern. Committees to investigate what are thought to be various areas of ineffectiveness in the industry have been set up. So have development groups, and an effort is being made by the Government to co-ordinate and encourage research into the industry with the aim of increasing its productivity and its effectiveness.

Summing Up

41. Consideration of the entries in the summarising table that have contemporary relevance, that is from position A onwards, makes it clear that at the present time the roles in the building industry are in a state of considerable confusion. The implications of this for the experience of any individual in the building team are, firstly, he finds that there is no settled and stable definition of what his job actually is, and secondly, nobody else can be clear about exactly what he does and what he is responsible for without finding out a lot more about the sort of building team he is in. The architect, the builder, the quantity surveyor, the sub-contractor, will be doing quite different jobs depending upon which of the many possible patterns of team structure they are currently operating in.

42. An architect, for example, may be a designer with limited power of decision for a package dealer. He may be operating in a negotiated contract and feel that "everybody seems to decide design" but himself, or he may be on a competitive contract for a technically relatively simple building and be almost completely free to determine design, as well as the structure of the building team. A builder may be a man who takes complete control of the whole building process as a package dealer and have all roles responsible to him. He may be in a negotiated contract and participate quite fully in design and in determining all the contractual arrangements. On the other hand, he may be working under a more traditional arrangement and find that he has to submit a competitive tender on the basis of a traditional bill of quantities, have a large part of the work he is responsible for done by sub-contractors not of his own choosing and be subject to the supervision of

the architect and the inquisition of the quantity surveyor.

43. So, too, with the quantity surveyor. He may be in a role restricted to the operation of the Standard Method of Measurement - as a technician only. He may be filling a more fully professional role and participating in the design stage with sophisticated techniques of estimating, and he may even be taking a decisive part in construction management through cost control advice to the builder.

44. As a result of this instability and lack of stable definitions of responsibility for members of the building team, there is a general anxiety among all concerned. This is understandable when from one project to the next a man may have no idea what his job is going to become. In this situation it is not surprising that relations between the various parties should be often strained and that tensions should exist, and this does in fact seem to be the case. As a result there is an understandable defensiveness on the part of everybody, particularly when entering a new relationship. In the absence of generally agreed rules for the relationship game, every man wants to ensure he is not a losing party. Natural developments of this are, on the one hand, the offensive/defensive stance that the corporate bodies representing the different roles tend to take up with each other, and on the other, a formal amiability that denies the underlying tensions.

45. As a part of our enquiries we put a small 'trial bore' into this area of attitudes and mutual perceptions in the building team. The results are reported in Appendix B. Although this was necessarily a very limited and tentative approach, it corroborates the general picture that emerges in this section. There do seem to be wide discrepancies in the social perceptions and the opinions about the value of contributions in the building process of each other among members of the building team. Indeed, it would seem that any communications in the building team are up against built-in difficulties before they start.

46. We do not want to leave the impression at this point that all is strife and difficulty with relations in the industry. We have been dealing with the general picture. Within this there are also genuine strivings for cohesion and co-operation. This study and the conference which is to receive it are largely the result of these positive forces.

47. In spite of the general picture that emerges, we hope that the considerations in this section have demonstrated that any lack of cohesion and co-ordination is less the result of ill-will or malignancy on the part of any groups or groups, but more the result of forces beyond the control of any individual or group and which are affecting all.

48. The way to improvement in these respects is not simple, wishing alone will not affect basic economic, social and technical forces. We would suggest that the first step would be to understand fully what are the nature and the effects of these forces currently operating both externally and internally. This analysis would become the starting point for developments towards generally agreed redefinitions of responsibilities and the stabilising of relationships which would allow for greater joint effectiveness. Many tools would be needed in such a job. One of the most valuable would be Operational Research, a tool that aims to disclose what operations any task actually consists of so that ways for achieving it more satisfactorily can be arrived at. In the next section this tool is described and its application to the problems of the industry is discussed.

TABLE EXEMPLIFYING THE DEVELOPMENT OF THE MAIN ROLES IN THE BUILDING TEAM AND THE RELATIONSHIPS BETWEEN THEM IN RESPONSE TO FORCES

OUTSIDE AND WITHIN THE INDUSTRY

FORCES DETERMINING FUNCTIONAL DIVISIONS AND ROLE RELATIONSHIPS		ROLES IN THE FUNCTIONAL AREAS OF THE BUILDING PROCESS		
External	Internal	Design Functions (Professional Roles)	Contract Area (Sub-Professional Roles)	Construction Functions (Commercial Roles)
Rise of bourgeois culture - great fire reconstruction	Need for design and single trade unit co-ordination	Emergence of Architect role Architect		Emergence of Independent commercial single trade units Brick-laying / Carpentry / Plumbing / etc.
Building demand of Industrial Revolution and Napoleonic Wars	Difficulties over architect/single trade unit payment agreements		Emergence of measurer role & 'measure & value' system	
Government takes action	Industry fails to meet demand			Establishment of Main Contractor role Sub-trader role emerges Main Contractor
	Need of basis for pre-agreement of contract price		Development of measuring from drawings -bill of quantities. Measurer role evolves to Quantity Surveyor role	
Technical development - Portland cement, steel, electricity, lifts, reinforced concrete, central heating, etc.				Emergence of specialist Sub-Contractor role Sub-Contractor Main Contractor
	Architect needs specialist design assistance	Emergence of role of Consultant & nominated Designer/Sub-Contractor Consultant / Designer/Sub-Contractor Architect		Nominated Sub-Contractor Main Contractor
Population growth - urban land more expensive - buildings become larger - contract/actual cost difference more significant - clients dissatisfied	Architect needs cost estimating assistance	.S. as ost Planner	Quantity Surveyors develop techniques of cost estimating (cost plan, etc) Emergence of QS in cost planner role. Become directly involved in decision-making, so fully professional	

Technical development - pre-stressed concrete, curtain walling, glass, aluminium, proprietary cladding system, prefabrication, etc.	Proportion of construction done by (particularly nominated supply and fix) sub-contractors increases			
War reconstruction, needs of full employment economy, large commercial development. Unit & overall costs high, more planning approvals, clients dissatisfied with delay/cost of traditional design and contracting procedures.	Building team members similarly dissatisfied, especially main contractors with proprietary interests		Emergence of the <u>negotiated contract</u> and <u>participation</u> by main contractor in design	Main Contractor
<u>POSITION A</u> Furthest point of consolidated development.		Q.S. as Cost Planner / Consultant / Designer/Sub-Contractor / Main Contractor as participant in design — Architect	QS as "standard method" measurer - for bill or "as made" (may not be involved in negotiated contract	Nominated Sub-Contractors / Sub-Contractors / Sub-Traders — Main Contractor
		<u>SOME CONTEMPORARY EMERGENT PATTERNS</u>		
Development of standard components/ modular design, prefabrication/industrialisation following models from other industries	Realisation by internal sponsors that larger, longer-term programmes than single job projects required to exploit developments	Roles as at Position A but modified by single co-ordination — e.g. County Architect	Emergence of <u>client/ design team consortia</u> <u>(CLASP, SCOLA, etc)</u> <u>serial contract</u>	Designated pre-fabricated components, nominated sub-contractors — Main Contractor
Client dissatisfied with delays, cost and confused responsibilities of traditional building team relationships. Believes single control of whole building process directly responsible to himself more efficient			Development of direct labour building	
	Main contractor believes low profit margins arise from pre-contract stages, common interest with dissatisfied client in overall project control		Emergence of <u>package</u> deal	
		Roles as at Position A but modified by single co-ordination	Direct labour client	or Package Dealer
Client doubts own competence as direct labour builder and dislikes being in the hands of the package dealer			Emergence of <u>Professional Contractor</u>	All work sub-contracted — Professional Contractor (Paid by fee)
Industry's productivity suspect, gets increasingly bad public image. Public pays for increasing proportion of industry's product. Government takes interest - sets up committees, development groups, research co-ordination	Divisions of functions between building team & patterns of relationship very various and unstable leading to tensions between individuals and groups. Many building team members also dissatisfied, impatient for change	?	?	?

<u>KEY:</u> ⏟ = range of responsibility of a role

--- = indicates a relationship of confused responsibility

SECTION IV

OPERATIONAL RESEARCH AND ITS APPLICATION TO THE BUILDING PROCESS*

What is O.R.?

1. O.R. is a scientific approach to the complex problems that arise in the direction and management of large systems of men, machines, materials and money in industry, business, government and defence. It is becoming increasingly difficult in a modern society to take decisions simply on the basis of commonsense, since there are many practical situations where there is a conflict of objectives, where the influence of external factors is obscure, and where accidental forces play an important part. Thus it is often not clear on what basis a decision should be taken or what factors enter into it. Operational Research is concerned with giving those whose job it is to take decisions the basis and information necessary for making these decisions as good as possible.

2. The first task of O.R. in any problem is to find out how the system works, the functions of its different parts, their interrelationships with each other, the main centres of control and co-ordination, and what information is necessary in order that this control be exercised. The resulting description is called a model of the system. It then remains to define an objective for the system as a whole - some index of performance. 'Output', 'cost/ton', 'net profit' are simple instances of indices of performance, but managers are usually concerned with more than one scale of performance and the often difficult job of finding some common link has to be undertaken. When this has been achieved the problem can be defined in O.R. terms: to adjust the factors within our control to achieve overall maximum performance (since this is achieved through a balancing of conflicting factors the term 'optimum' and the verb 'to optimise' are frequently used, see paragraphs II/14 and II/21). Various techniques, depending on the problem, exist for solution of problems defined in this way. When an answer has been found it must be tested in practice, modified

---

* We would like to acknowledge the valuable assistance we have had from Dr. Eric Totman, a member of the Operational Research Society, in preparing this section.

if necessary, and so on. Thus the approach of O.R. is quantitative, observational, and experimental. It is therefore scientific in the full sense, but with its interest centred on human objectives. It is concerned not simply with finding out in a detached way how things work, but how this knowledge can be used to achieve practical objectives - O.R. is 'involved' or committed'.

3. In the attempt to optimise performance, O.R. is led to consider what will happen when the social structure implied in the model takes different forms. Some forms of organisation will be more effective, and will contribute more to better performance (on whatever criterion) than will others. Such an issue as centralised versus decentralised production or sales organisation is familiar in manufacturing industry. This is the 'organisational variable' which is discussed further in paragraph 26.

4. Operational Research can be used not merely to predict the optimum behaviour of existing man/machine systems, but to forecast by mathematical techniques the behaviour of systems conceived to be organised in an entirely different way. Clearly some assumptions have always to be built into such hypothetical exercises, which require, in accordance with normal scientific procedure, that testing in practice is necessary. Such an approach does, however, allow the investigator to think constructively and quantitatively about complicated matters.

O.R. and the Building Process

5. We now consider how this approach can be applied to the building process. Looking at any building process we can distinguish three main functions. Two are obvious: design and contruction. The third will be called co-ordination. Co-ordination is almost equivalent in meaning to 'control', 'planning' or 'management', but is more descriptive of the relating together of separate activities and their concerted direction towards a common purpose. The co-ordination function bears an analagous relationship to the remaining two functions as the central nervous system does to the physical activities of the body. In the building process, the different members of the building team all have a role with respect to this function, but in the conventional case one member has a more central position and there is a change of roles at the contract stage. Thus, it is the architect who exercises the main co-ordinating function before the

contract is signed, and the builder afterwards.

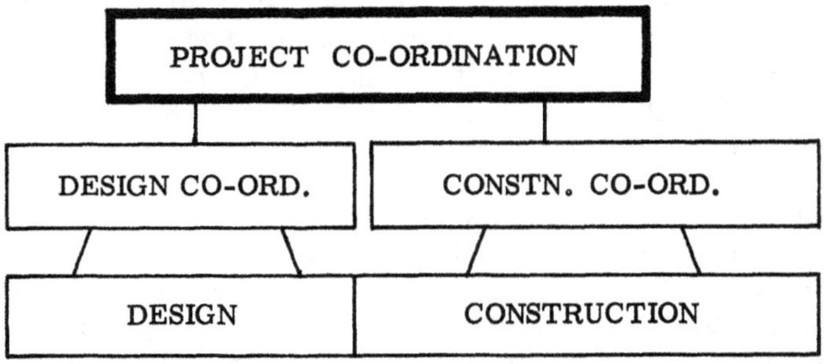

When the builder assumes responsibility for construction, some of the members of the existing team, for example sub-contractors and the quantity surveyor, have to fit into a new pattern of relationships, based on the builder and subject to his co-ordination function. Others remain closely associated with the architect, consultants for example.

6. All three functions are activated by the agency of communication in some form. To study communications with a view to suggesting practical improvements involves studying the relationships between the members of the building team, the communications which these relationships imply, and which of the three functions these communications serve. Since we are concerned with improvement, some criterion or measure of performance must be defined, and all variables involved in the building process, including organisational variables, related to it. (These points are discussed further in paragraph 26.)

7. The above, then, is a brief description of the role of O.R. and its manner of approach to the communication problem. We now consider what specific problems and technqiues seem likely to help in this.

8. The first problem is to decide what is the measure of performance with respect to which improvement may be assessed? Considering the building process as a whole, three factors come immediately to mind: time, cost (the outlay of the client) and goodness of design. Time is related to cost in that the builder's price is related to time, however variable this relationship may be. Before the construction phase, time has a relationship to the consumption of professional services. 'Goodness of design' has aesthetic and functional elements. These are difficult to quantify in view of their subjective nature, although the problem

is a legitimate one: how much additional effort is worthwhile in continuing to improve design in an aesthetic sense? The functional aspects concerns how well the design will serve its purpose. Part of this problem is akin to the aesthetic one, but the rest is economic. If a building is bad in design, then high repairs and maintenance charges and the less obvious costs of user inconvenience will be entailed in future, representing a charge at 'present value' to the client (the money to be set aside now which at compound interest will grow to the expected extra cost). This is highly theoretical, in view of the lack of data on such matters, but is mentioned to show that 'goodness of design' has a cost component as well as subjective elements.

9. 'Cost' is put forward as a tentative first approach to a criterion of performance for the building process. There is, however, an important distinction between the sense in which it is usually used (client's outlay) and what is intended here. What is meant here is a direct measure of the consumption of all resources, professional time, builder's outlay, client's expected future repairs and maintenance bill (discounted) and so on. (This is comparable with the situation in a large industrial firm which designs and executes work for itself - there is no confusion here as to whose money is involved). The relationship between time and cost (in this sense) during the design stage is probably complex. A very short time for design may result in a bad building. However, our work leads us to suppose that with design effort remaining the same, the time involved is greatly affected by relationships between members of the building team so that a material reduction in design time could take place without deterioration in other respects and hence reduce costs. (Paragraph 23 will illustrate the possibilities here.) The matter requires careful detailed study. However, it is suggested as a crude approximation that optimising the whole building process will consist in reducing the time of the design function and minimising the cost (to the builder) of the construction function - under normal practice this reduced cost can only be passed on to the client if the builder can foresee, with some accuracy, what this will be. Minimisation of cost has the implication that the productivity of professional and industrial labour is increased.

The Critical Path Method *

10. We now consider the techniques necessary for the task. It must be emphasised that the examples given in the following are illustrative,

* See p. 60

not the results of research. They are intended to indicate a way of thinking about the problem and the direction in which it may lead.

11. What is required is a frame in which to represent the whole building process. One of these is supplied by the Critical Path Method. In this a building process is regarded as a network reflecting the interdependence in time of the tasks and decisions it comprises. Some definitions are necessary·

An activity is a task or operation which has to be performed and which requires time, e.g. preparing drawings, estimating material requirements etc.

An event is a recognisable stage in the programme, such as receipt of material, arrival of equipment, completion of drawings, and occurs at a point in time and is considered to have no duration.

A network is a flow chart made up of one or more series of events joined by activity lines to depict their interdependencies and inter-relationships.

Any project can be regarded as comprising a network of 'events' and 'activities'.

Let us consider the following simple network:

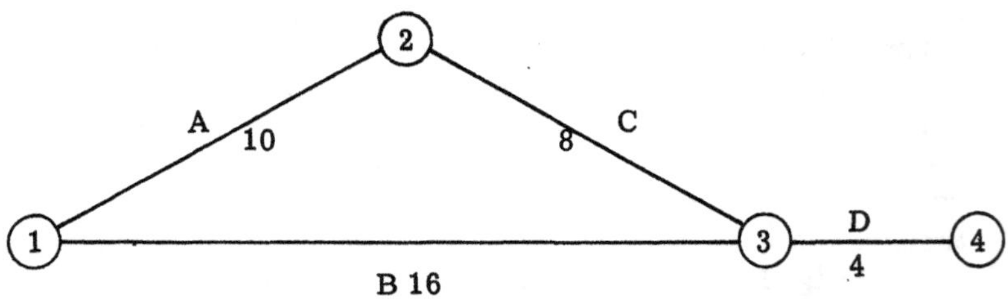

* It would appear to us now (December 1964), having been engaged in the major investigation for just over a year, that the apparent emphasis here on the critical path method is somewhat excessive. In particular, the design process requires a sharper form of analysis then this method - a production tool - can provide. Our further study has also suggested that the critical path method (as distinct from network analyses) may be less appropriate to the control of construction activities than we originally supposed. With these reservations, we feel the account given on pages 64 - 66 of these techniques offers a useful indication of the possible value they may have in providing a starting point for developing improved forms of collaboration between the parties concerned.

FIG. IV 1.

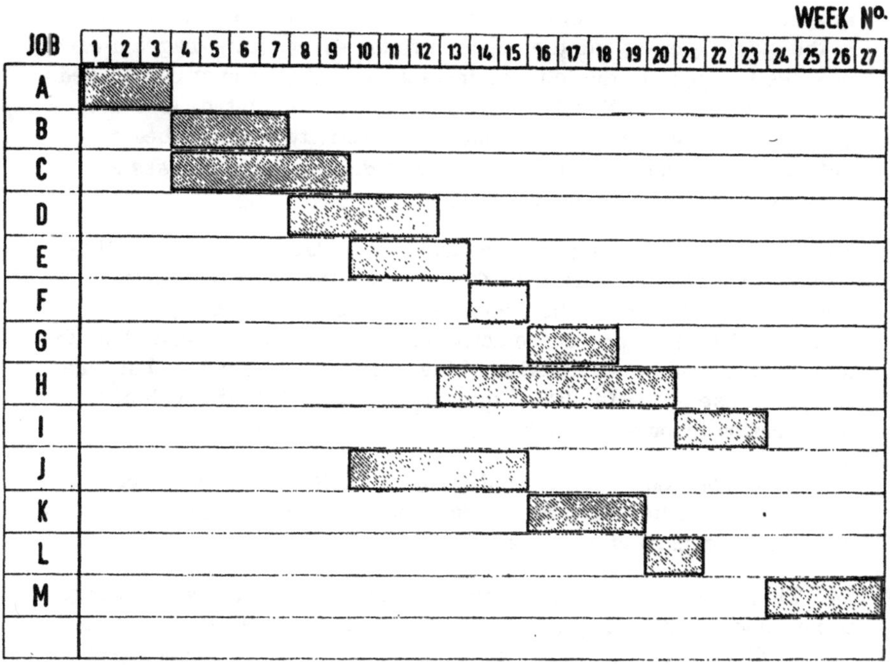

FIG. IV 2.

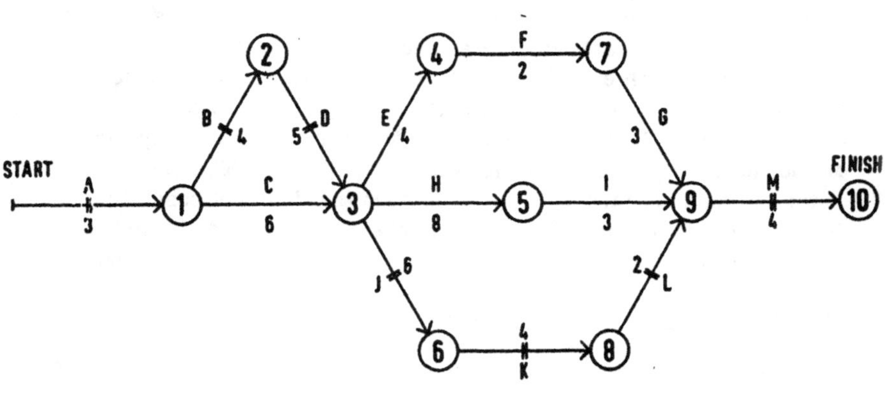

The starting event is denoted by (1) and the finish event by (4.) There are four activities A, B, C and D. An activity is generally referred to by its starting event number/finish event number, e.g. activity A is activity (1)-(2) and is represented by an arrow the tail of which is the starting event and the head the finish event. The diagram expresses the logic of the job, for instance event (3) cannot be reached until the three activities A, B and C have been completed, also activities A and B can run concurrently, and activity C cannot begin until activity A has been completed. The diagram summarises a number of statements about relationships.

12. Something more is required, and that is durations of the activities. If A = 10 (days), B = 16, C = 8, D = 4 then it is obvious that the whole project cannot be completed in less than 22 days, i.e. (A + C + D). If any of the activities A, C or D take longer than the stated time then the completion of the project will be delayed accordingly. These activities lie on the critical path. It is the path of longest duration through the network.

13. A simple example of a small project made up of jobs of specified duration is indicated by the Bar Chart in Figure IV.1. It is required to construct a network.

14. This is done by starting with the first job A and drawing an arrow to represent it (the length of arrow does not represent the job duration). The tail of the arrow will represent start time or zero (see Figure IV.2). The head of the arrow represents the completion of the first job. From event (1) other arrows representing jobs B and C are drawn; these start as soon as job A is complete. From the head of job B, event (2), another arrow emanates representing the job D which may not begin until job B is completed. This process is continued until the project is complete. The best time estimates obtainable are associated with each job and the critical path is found by determining the longest time path through the project network. The jobs on this path are critical and cannot be reduced in time except by the use of additional resources of manpower or equipment. The critical path of the network is marked ||. It is seen that it is not possible to determine from the Bar Chart which jobs are critical and which are not, and herein lies a great advantage of the critical path diagram.

How does the Critical Path Method Work?

15. For the co-ordination function to proceed at all adequately a com-

plete grasp of the project is obviously most important. Only by understanding the system can co-ordination achieve minimum time, minimum cost projects.

16. Normally when building is held up due to bad weather, labour difficulties or late deliveries of materials, to speed up the project everyone involved in the process is put onto overtime. In fact, only 'critical jobs' need to put on to full overtime and overtime need only be applied to non-critical jobs to keep pace with the accelerated schedule of the critical jobs. In this way the project is speeded up as fast as possible, but with the expenditure of the minimum amount of money.

17. The method can be used initially to give indications of the costs of various degrees of project acceleration and to indicate to management whether an accelerated schedule is worth while.

18. Suppose the completion date of a building can be advanced by three months at an additional cost of £60,000 on critical jobs. If the indirect costs a month are £25,000 there will be a net saving of £15,000 on the project; this may not be enough, but if a large income is obtained more quickly by the fact that the building is in commission three months sooner than otherwise, this will have a bearing on the decision.

19. Those jobs not on the critical path are called 'floaters', that is, there is more time available to complete the job than is necessary, e.g. activity B in paragraph 11 has two days float. If the critical path is too long, it can be shortened by the application of overtime, extra manpower etc., without requiring an acceleration in most of the 'floater' jobs. In the case of large scale projects this saving can be large in terms of avoiding the use of unnecessary manpower, equipment, etc. By a further extension of the method, it is possible to use the critical path concept for smoothing labour requirements, determining expediting costs, for inter-project manpower loading and equipment scheduling, etc.

20. For small projects it is possible to use the Critical Path Method without the use of a computer, however for large projects with a high number of jobs (e.g. greater than 500 activities) a computer is necessary. Projects which need to be updated frequently will normally require a computer.

21. Some other points about the Critical Path Method are:

(a) As the project proceeds the full effects of any delays on the rest of the project can be estimated.

(b) It allows of better co-ordination between the key people.

(c) It makes possible economy in management resources by focussing management thought, skill and decision onto those activities which are, or are likely to be, in difficulties.

(d) It facilitates the handover to new management in 'mid-stream'.

22. Let us now apply the Critical Path Method to the preconstruction phase (without entering into any degree of detail). We are concerned with minimising the pre-construction time (and hence cost). The following example is based on "Pre-contract Practice" by the Aqua Group (4).

Activities	Events	Time (estimates)
	1. Client decides to build	-
A. Client consults with architect	2. Architect is appointed	1 week
B. Prepare sketch plan and cost plan	3. Sketch and cost plan complete	4 weeks
C. Consideration of plan by client and revision	4. Approval obtained	4 weeks
D. Outline approvals obtained	5. Plan approved	4 weeks
E. Working drawings prepared	6. Working drawings complete	12 weeks
F. Consultants prepare drawings	7. Consultants' drawings complete	7 weeks
G. Specialist requirements considered and requirements stated.	8. Complete specialist requirements	3 weeks

Activities	Events	Time (estimates)
H. Prepare bills of quantities	9. Bills of quantities complete	4 weeks
I. Tendering out	10. Replies of tenders received	4 weeks
J. Tenders considered	11. Tender selected	2 weeks
K. Contract drawn up	12. Contract signed	1 week
L. Builder prepares	13. Site work commences	6 weeks

The simple network is given in Fig. IV. 3.

N. B. (a) The critical path is (1) - (2) - (3) - (5) - (6) - (9) - (10) - (11) - (12) - (13) and is 38 weeks duration.

(b) Activities are given by the start and finish event numbers, e.g. activity F is (5) - (7).

(c) Figures in the square represent the earliest event time and the figures in the circle the latest event time.

(d) Event (4) has four weeks 'float'. Event (7) has six weeks 'float' (22 - 16 = 6 weeks). Float is latest event time minus earliest event time. This means that activity F can be completed at any time between 16 and 22 weeks after the start event (1) without affecting the finish event (13) time.

23. Now if one has a negotiated contract with a builder it is possible to introduce him as a member of the team at an earlier stage than event (12) in the above network, in fact he can enter at event (5). The network is now given in Fig. IV. 4. The advantages are as follows

(a) The pre-construction phase can be completed more quickly (25 weeks instead of 38 weeks).

(b) The builder has the chance to communicate in the early stages with the architect and other specialists, including the nominated sub-contractors, (after week 9 instead of week 32).

(c) The builder can order his materials earlier, and also set up his construction network of building activities. The builder can allocate his known resources of equipment and manpower by trade - the latter is especially important where the builder may have work going on in several places.

24. It may be possible to go further and introduce the consultants, the quantity surveyor, and also the sub-contractors at an early stage so that free discussion between all members of the team can take place at the design stage, so enabling them to start their work earlier. For example, activity E (prepare the working drawings) might be split into three parts. After completion of Working Drawings I, the Bills of Quantities I are prepared, and while these are being prepared, Working Drawings II can be prepared concurrently. Similarly for specialist design work. The network will now appear in the form given in Fig. IV. 5.

25. The preceding illustrates how the Critical Path Method could be employed for studying the potential advantages of different types of team-structure. In the form given here it does not necessarily show what communications are taking place between the members of the building team, but the network presentation could be used for any building process to show the patterns of exchange of information between members through all its phases. This requires careful detailed investigation. It would be of interest to see, for example, how much 'to-ing and fro-ing' there is between members at a particular stage and what form this takes. This could affect the time on the process critical path and also highlight techniques of communication that could be improved. A detailed consideration of all the techniques of communication, formal and informal, is of course vital to any full-scale study, but this must obviously be undertaken with co-operation of persons representative of the building team within the general O. R. /sociological framework given here.

Other Techniques - An Approach to the Problem of Co-ordination

26. It is evident that the Critical Path Method has two potentialities, one as a means of investigation of functional relationships and communications, and the other as a tool of the co-ordinating function itself. This raises the critical organisational variable problem of who, or what group, should exercise this function. This calls for both detailed O.R. studies of the many operations involved as well

FIG. IV 3.

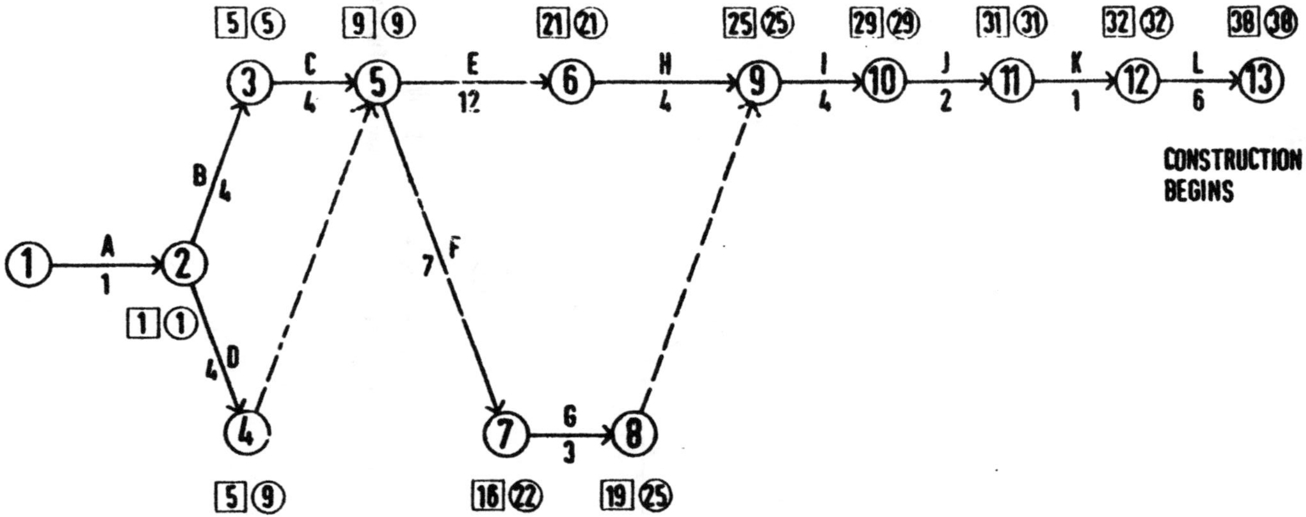

FIG. IV 4.

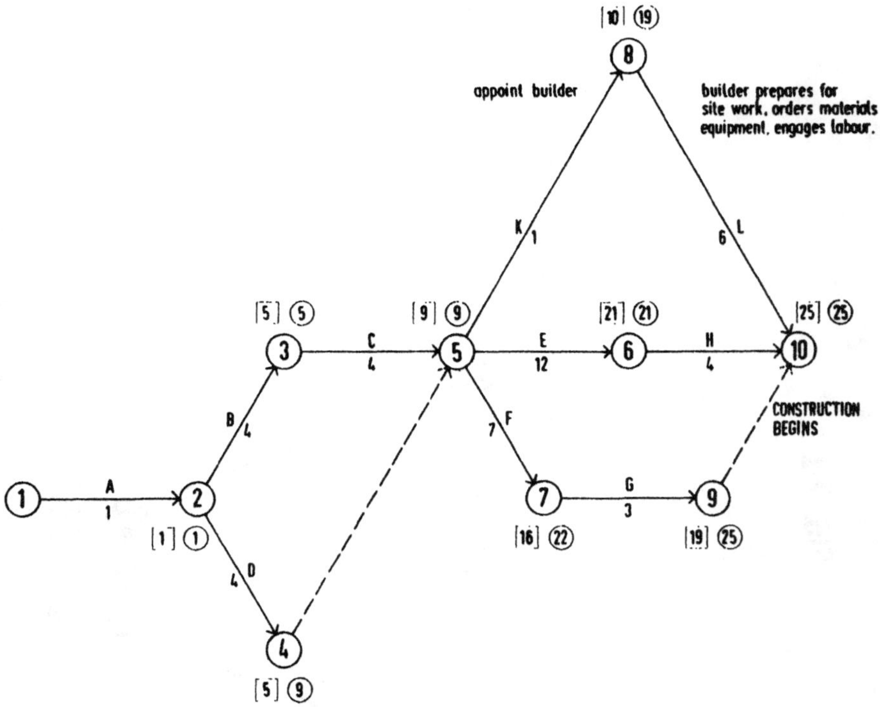

N.B. 1. the times used are the same as in Fig. IV 3.

2. the event numbers are not the same as in Fig. IV 3.

FIG. IV 5.

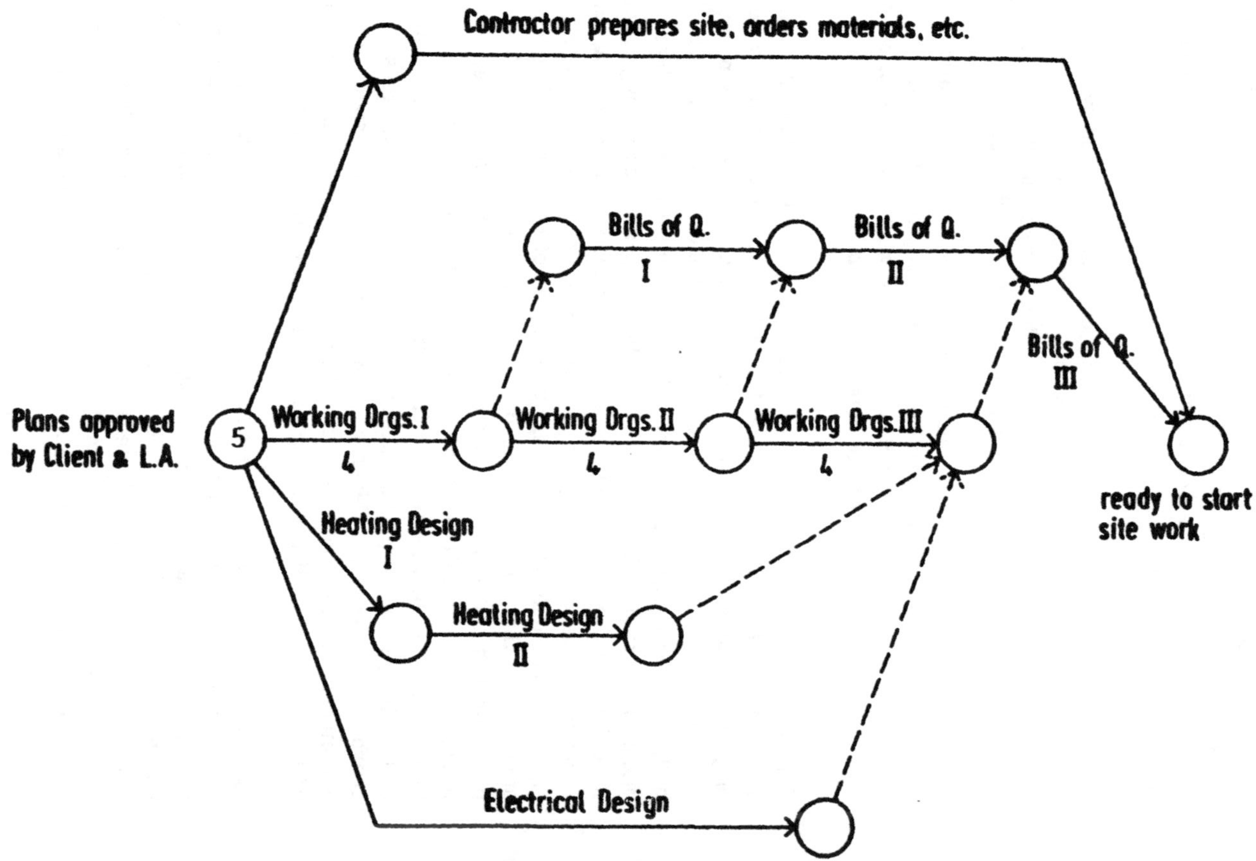
Contractor prepares site, orders materials, etc.
Plans approved by Client & L.A.
5
Working Drgs. I
4
Working Drgs. II
4
Working Drgs. III
4
Bills of Q. I
Bills of Q. II
Bills of Q. III
Heating Design I
Heating Design II
Electrical Design
ready to start site work

as rigorous analysis of the historical, social and present 'political' forces operating among the existing building team roles with their special interests, professional as well as commercial. Two hypotheses may, however, be put forward:

Hypothesis 1: that a co-ordinating function exercised over both design and construction functions by a single person (or group) is better than one where the functions have a different co-ordinator.

Hypothesis 2: that if design and construction functions must have separate co-ordinators, then the best system of this kind is one where there is an early exchange of relevant information.

27. Whatever form the pattern of relationships may take for the construction function, it is clear that the critical path technique may be of great use to whoever has the main co-ordinating role. The person who now fills this role, which could be called the 'construction controller', is the main contractor. His responsibilities include both planning the project before work is undertaken, and controlling it once it begins. In the planning stage he is concerned with determining what resources of labour and equipment are necessary to minimise cost, and this technique could be a very useful part of his work. We understand in fact that some builders do use versions of it already. Once the project is under way discrepancies from the plan will arise, both in regard to time and cost, and the means must be found for bringing them to light so that remedial action can be taken. For large projects, elaborate systems of management reporting based on computers are in course of development. Much remains to be done with respect to small and medium scale work to see that the same principles can be applied with the simplicity that the practical situation would require.

28. Situations will often arise where the construction controller's resources allocation problem is complicated by competitive demands for the same type of manpower or equipment. This can happen on repetitive housing projects (48) or with respect to a single contractor with more than one project. It is because of the effect of accidental factors, e.g. weather, and variations in the time taken to complete the same job, that a congestion problem may arise. In recent years queueing

theory has developed which gives new insight into these problems.* Further, the existence of computers allows for the possibility of testing, for example, what the effect is of different allocations of equipment or labour forces in given trades upon delays and production rates. Such an exercise - paper experimentation - is called simulation and is widely used in O.R. for complex problems of this kind. Such matters may seem a little remote from the communication problem, but its relevance can be seen when one considers that such matters have a vital bearing on the co-ordination function in the construction phase and the relationship between all parties involved in it.

29. The approach to organisation given here has been empirical. Two hypotheses have been put forward on the basis of what might be called 'ordinary commonsense'. These refer to only one aspect of the building team - the co-ordination function. In indicating ways in which an improvement in the building process might be effected, by bringing all concerned with design into relationship with each other at an early stage, the approach is similar. Is there a systematic way of dealing with organisational variables, more in accordance with the approach of O.R. in other spheres? There is good reason to suppose that one can be developed from the interest that exists in this subject and the presence of conceptual tools in the social sciences with an obvious bearing upon it. What is needed, among other things, is a means of placing a 'rating' on the importance of a role at different points in the process (e.g. the architect during the design phase, or the builder during the construction phase), and a measure of the 'strength' of relationship between one member of the team and another (how closely interdependent are their functions?). From considerations such as these, ways of optimising organisational structure may be suggested which can then be tested against practical experience and experiment. It might be found in the case of the building process

---

* Queueing theory is sometimes called congestion theory. It is concerned with the manner in which a service facility (a man/machine system) of known capacity, copes with jobs (or 'customers') that arrive in a random or a partly-random manner. It is concerned with calculating such things as: length of queue, average waiting time, the effects of increased or diminished service facilities.

that certain types of process called for one type of organisation pattern and other processes for other patterns.

Summing Up

30. (1) The general approach of O.R. to the communication problem involves the setting up of criteria of performance against which improvement can be measured. The defining of appropriate criteria is a matter of gradual evolution, but 'cost' may be taken as a starting point.

(2) The building process is regarded as the development of and the relationship among three functions: design, construction and co-ordination.

(3) Techniques exist which enable processes to be studied as networks of activities and events.

(4) Such networks give an insight into ways in which the logic may be changed to effect an improvement. Such changes in logic have organisational and communication implications.

(5) The critical path technique has considerable potentialities for improving the co-ordination function.

(6) There is a need for more 'carry-over' in the co-ordination function with respect to design and construction phases. This requires detailed investigation. Two hypotheses are advanced.

(7) Fundamental research is needed to quantify roles in terms of their relative effects on the inter-dependent operations of the building process and the inevitable relationships between roles this gives rise to.

PART TWO

PROBLEMS, RECOMMENDATIONS, AND REQUIREMENTS

PROBLEMS

From our study we consider the following to be the main problems associated with communications in the building industry. Of the five problems outlined below, the first two affect in some degree all members of the building team. The third mainly affects architects and consultants. The fourth again affects all members, but mainly quantity surveyors, while the fifth mainly affects builders, sub-contractors and those on the supply side. We consider the first two to be of equal importance to the others. They concern the making and development of relations with the most crucial part of the industry's environment - those whom it exists to serve.

1. COMMUNICATION WITH PROSPECTIVE CLIENTS

ARE THOSE WHO MUST TAKE THE KEY DECISIONS ABOUT SPENDING £3,000 MILLION A YEAR ON BUILDING SUFFICIENTLY AWARE OF ALL THE SERVICES THE INDUSTRY HAS TO OFFER TO BE ABLE TO DIRECT THEIR SPENDING MOST ADVANTAGEOUSLY?

Building is a service industry, it makes specific things to customer's order. But many prospective customers do not know enough of the range of technical and professional services available to them to decide their orders satisfactorily, or to make the first approach to the industry which is appropriate to their needs. Those who take building decisions are not randomly scattered in the population. The industry could do much to help by identifying its most likely customers and communicating to them information about itself.

2. COMMUNCIATIONS BETWEEN CLIENTS AND ADVISERS

TO WHAT EXTENT DOES ANY MEMBER OF THE BUILDING TEAM CALLED UPON TO ADVISE A CLIENT FIND OUT ALL ABOUT HIS NEEDS AND ABOUT ALL THE POSSIBILITIES THAT THE INDUSTRY CAN OFFER HIM?

How often does a client (individual or corporate) find that had he known as much at the beginning of a project as he knows at the end, he would have made quite different initial decisions? There is seldom a complete enough exploration of all the client's needs and of the limitations he must accept - nor is he sufficiently informed of all the possible means of meeting his needs. The matching of needs and possibilities is seldom fully achieved, so the brief can rarely be adequate and clearly understood by all. This can lead to difficulties and reduced efficiency at all subsequent stages of the project.

3. COMMUNICATIONS WITHIN THE DESIGN TEAM

THE EFFECTIVE ACHIEVEMENT OF THE COMMON DESIGN TASK REQUIRES FULL, RAPID, AND CONTINUOUS INTERCHANGE OF INFORMATION. WHY DOES THIS NOT OCCUR?

Sufficient thought and time does not seem to be given to ensuring, either as a design team brief or during the designing process, that all who must contribute understand the common objective similarly and fully. There is seldom a full awareness of all the steps necessary to realise an optimum overall outcome without loss of time, and the means of ensuring design co-ordination is often not clear. If the intercommunication problems of the design team were analysed in operational terms, more effective and rapid techniques could be devised for solving them.

4. COMMUNICATIONS RELATED TO CONTRACT

THE INFORMATION EXCHANGED AS A BASIS FOR ENTERING INTO CONTRACTUAL OBLIGATIONS IS WIDELY EXPERIENCED BY ALL AS INADEQUATE. WHY IS THIS SO?

There is a very wide and very complex variety of ways in which the members of the building team can be contractually related to each other. But when a contract is entered into it is unusual for any of those concerned to know with any degree of certainty just what he can expect of others, and what others will expect of him. The nature of relationships is defined afresh for everybody as any project develops at the price of delays and confusions. The frank sorting out of these difficulties at the commencement of a contract is prevented by the silent reservations of all parties about points of possible disadvantage each feels he must watch for.

5. COMMUNICATIONS WITHIN THE CONSTRUCTION TEAM

CONTROL OF CONSTRUCTION REQUIRES:

(a) EFFECTIVE COMMUNICATION WITHIN THE CONSTRUCTION TEAM, AND

(b) EFFECTIVE COMMUNICATIONS BETWEEN THE CONSTRUCTION TEAM AND OTHERS.

HOW OFTEN ARE THESE CONDITIONS REALISED?

The basic decisions of construction control are often incomplete or unduly rushed because necessary information is not available sufficiently ahead of time, or is not complete enough. On many occasions members of the construction team could, but do not, ease this problem by supplying the data that would facilitate the preparation of fuller and more useful information by others. Building construction is remarkable among industrial activities for the lack of detailed information about how it proceeds. Until more is known there can be no basis for improvement.

RECOMMENDATIONS AND REQUIREMENTS

If building is thought of without the people involved it can be seen as a chain of interdependent operations - briefing, designing, estimating, billing, manufacturing, supplying, assembling, etc. To undertake these operations a wide variety of resources of material and skill is required, and must be co-ordinated.

To study the building process as a series of interlocked operations requiring the application of many resources leads to the setting up of models for improving it.

The resources remain under the control of people and organisations whom we have called 'resource controllers'. The main difficulties in communications have to do with the relationships between resource controllers.

The central problem arises from the fact that the basic relationship which exists among resource controllers has the character of interdependent autonomy. There is a lack of match between the technical interdependence of the resources and the organisational independence of those who control them.

In Section III of Part One we have said something of how the present situation in this respect has come about, and have taken a brief look at the forces both inside and outside the industry which affect it.

For three centuries the industry has been struggling to reconcile technical interdependence and organisational independence. This struggle has not been made easier by the alternating impatience or indifference of society, according to the high or low level of demand for the industry's services, and by the need of the industry to absorb technical developments and to find a role for new resource controllers. We suggest that the industry need not continue to be controlled only by the forces acting on it externally and internally. Knowledge and techniques in Operational Research and the Social Sciences now exist, which allow the industry to assert something of its own control over these forces.

Any attempt to re-order the division of responsibilities among resource controllers that might arise from a purely technical study would very soon run up against deep-seated difficulties of conflicting values and vested professional, technical and commercial interests. These often represent the commitments of a lifetime, and demand respect. We would therefore suggest concurrent studies of:

(a) the pattern of interlocking operations involved in the building process, what these are and how they might be improved;

(b) the nature of the distinctive competence vested in the existing resource controller roles, how these relate to each other, and how these relationships in turn match with the technical relatedness of the resources each controls.

The outcome of these dual studies would be the setting up of models, initially on a limited scale, that could point the way towards improvements. The results of these studies would, by agreement, be quickly made available to the whole industry.

Applied research along these lines would need several conditions. First, the early stages of such studies must be undertaken within specific units in the industry; for example, one design office, one building project, one building site. Second, they must be under conditions of experimental protection - i.e. there must be willingness by all those immediately involved to try something new. This condition is not possible unless the research is done within a relationship of professional confidentiality - nothing is reported without the agreement of those who have been involved. Third, the situations in which these studies are undertaken and the models developed and tested under real-life conditions must not be too different from those normally found in the industry. A laboratory is needed, but a real-life laboratory that is recognisably the same kind of situation as is usual - if a little different in some particulars.

There are many new techniques and systems of building developing throughout the country. There are also new patterns of relationships emerging among resource contollers - professional consortia, all-in services, and design team/client consortia etc. Such growing points as these, and others like them, can provide the research sites both for model building and testing their efficiency under conditions of action.

<u>We recommend</u> that research be undertaken on the basis of protected experiments into the interdependent operations of the building process concurrently with studies of the roles and relationships of the building team members involved.

<u>The objects</u> of the research would be:

1. to develop models for improving both operations and relationships;
2. to test the value of these models in real-life conditions;
3. to disseminate information about them and assist in their wider application and further development.

The work recommended could not become a possibility unless several conditions were met.

Such a project would need some widely-based body to take responsibility for financing, commissioning and steering it, as the NJCC has done for this pilot study. We believe that if the industry as a whole is to accept and support the research, a body more broadly based than the NJCC will be found necessary.

At many points within and related to the industry, research projects are under way. We refer not only to the work going on at the Building Research Station, in the various Research Associations, and at Manchester College of Science and Technology, etc., but also to that being undertaken by various bodies within the industry. A study of contract procedures is being made by the Quantity Surveyors' Committee of the RICS; a study of construction management roles is being made by the Board of Building Education at the IOB; the RIBA has formulated projects for the study of architects' drawings and for research into the impact of the industrialisation of building on the profession;

the NCBMP is contemplating a technical catalogue for architects' use, and there must be many others. We would therefore suggest that a census of present and contemplated research projects should be made. Much more could be gained from all these separate research efforts, and overlapping avoided, if there were some form of co-ordination among them.

<u>We recommend</u> that an industry-wide representative body should be developed:

1. to take responsibility for a research project as recommended;
2. in parallel with this research project, to initiate a census of present and contemplated researches in the industry, and to develop a means of co-ordinating them.

Our terms of reference require us to give some indication of the resources which would be required for any research arising from our recommendations. Obviously, this will depend on how much it is decided should be undertaken, and on the resources made available. We recommend below what we consider to be the minimum requirements to allow an effective start to be made. This covers only resources from outside the industry. Effective applied research will require these resources to be combined with others from within the industry, mainly from those in the research sites where the work will be done. Their knowledge and ideas and access to the information they control will be necessary, but most important will be their willingness to co-operate in testing developing models.

The initial direct outlay we recommend involves a sum representing 0.0007 per cent of the industry's annual turnover. We see it only as a bridging operation - work on a much larger scale will be needed if the industry is to take a significant part in determining its own future development and progressively improving its performance.

<u>We recommend</u> that to make an effective start on communications research a team of three or four research staff plus supporting statistical and secretarial services would be required over a period of about eighteen months. We would expect this to require funds of approximately £20,000.

APPENDICES

APPENDIX A

EXTRACT FROM MEMORANDUM 32M CONSIDERED BY THE NATIONAL JOINT CONSULTATIVE COMMITTEE ON 12TH OCTOBER 1962

Third Report from Sub-committee on Communications in the Building Industry.

3. Pilot Study and Conference

3.1. A pilot study is recommended:

a) because the scope and form of the major project cannot be defined by the committee: it is too large and complex a question. The pilot study will have as its main objective the definition of terms of reference for the major project and an estimate of the resources needed to mount it;

b) a pilot study is in the tradition of Tavistock's work (see Attachment 2). It will also show how far the major project is viable and enable the parties to withdraw without much loss if it seems impracticable;

c) the conference will enable a cross-section of the industry to become involved in and committed to the major project. This is essential, for the NJCC alone would not command sufficient allegiance to ensure that the recommendations of the major project were fully implemented. If the leaders of the industry can hear the results of the pilot survey, criticise them and approve terms of reference for the main study, real success is much more likely.

3.2. The pilot study will not only set out to define the major project. It will be a significant contribution to the communications problem in its own right. At the least Tavistock/Operational Research see it as providing an analysis of the whole complex of building industry communications in scientific terms and in relation to similar problems elsewhere in industry: not a course of treatment, but a diagnosis. It may even be that the new description will lead to a new understanding and to new attitudes which will make changes in the pattern of communications seem more sensible and more acceptable.

3.3. The pilot study would be undertaken by Tavistock/Operational Research staff advised by a steering committee. There would be no staff from the industry working on the pilot study. In the main study it is tentatively thought that two Tavistock/Operational Research men would be assisted by two men seconded from the industry.

4. Tavistock/Operational Research Society

4.1. The first report made the point that none of the three constituent bodies should act as a base for the research. Since then, and after discussions with experienced people outside the industry, the sub-committee has been convinced that the research base must be entirely neutral if the project is to be successful. In addition it must have powerful expert resources on which to draw.

4.2. The sub-committee has considered three University Departments, the Building Research Station and Tavistock/Operational Research as research bases. The Departments of Architecture at the Universities of Durham and London are from their nature not fully neutral and therefore have not been followed up. The third, Manchester College of Technology, is already committed to directing the study of the economy and structure of the Building Industry to be financed by DSIR, and could not take charge of another major project.

4.3. BRS while very anxious to assist in making the project a success did not feel it would itself provide a satisfactory base:

a) because there are serious administrative difficulties in accommodating non-civil servants on a government establishment;

b) because BRS wants to see another growing point for building industry research established. It considers the industry badly needs a non-official research interest and sees the NJCC project as a possible starting point.

4.4. Quite apart from these negative indications, the Tavistock Institute/Operational Research approach seems to the sub-committee to have substantial advantages. The Tavistock Institute is in the process of setting up a unit (probably to be called The Operational Research Institute)* in combination with the Operational Research Society. It is to be a non-profit making research institute devoted to widening the applications of Operational Research, particularly in fields where the social sciences are involved; and in developing the theory and methodology of Operational Research. Like the Tavistock Institute it will operate by doing pure research as well as undertaking field work as consultants on behalf of clients.

4.5. Tavistock/Operational Research will certainly be neutral. They will be able to tackle the communications problem with a combination of disciplines. The Tavistock Institute has for many years acted as adviser on personnel matters to Unilever and has conducted much research on its behalf; it has done extensive research work in engineering and in coal mining, and is currently acting as research consultants to the Technical University of Norway on a project concerned with the development of "industrial democracy", jointly sponsored by the Norwegian Confederation of Employers and the Norwegian Trades Unions. Operational Research, of course, is a discipline which is widely used throughout industry and government, especially by defence departments.

4.6. The Tavistock/Operational Research staff concerned are keenly interested in the NJCC project and see it as exactly the kind of problem their new unit is meant to tackle. They are prepared to undertake a pilot study without any certainty that the main project will follow, and they are prepared to make staff available from November - March next. The two men directly concerned are Dr. G.W. Higgin of Tavistock and Mr. Neil Jessop of the Operational Research Society. (Attachment 1 gives details about Tavistock Operational Research and their staff: Attachment 2 describes their approach to the project).

---

* This is now finalised. The new unit is to be The Institute for Operational Research (Tavistock Institute). It officially comes into being on 1st May 1963, and its first director is to be Mr. Neil Jessop.

4.7. Nevertheless it must be realised that an element of risk is involved in this proposal. These disciplines have not been much involved with building industry research in the past and have not previously combined to study so large and complex an industry as building. (Though Professor Mace and the Medical Research Council used similar techniques in a small study of building workers in 1946-48). This is an additional reason for a pilot study. The view of outsiders consulted by the sub-committee is that there is a high probability of success and that Tavistock have a very high reputation in industry.

Attachment 1

THE TAVISTOCK INSTITUTE OF HUMAN RELATIONS

AND THE OPERATIONAL RESEARCH SOCIETY

The Tavistock Institute describes its function as the study of human relations in conditions of well-being, conflict or breakdown, in the family, the work-group and the larger organisation.

The Institute works in two divisions. One is concerned with family and social psychiatry and is medically orientated. The other, with which the NJCC would deal, is concerned with organisations and their behaviour, and with social change. Here it conducts its research in collaboration with, and often as a consultant to, private and public bodies, trains personnel for such work, and offers advisory services.

The Institute was incorporated in 1947 as a company limited by guaran tee and not for profit. It is managed by a Council of which Sir Hugh Beaver is at present Chairman. Other members include Professor Phelps Brown, Professor of Economics of Labour at London University and a member of the National Economic Development Council, Professor W.R. Hawthorne, Professor of Applied Thermodynamics at Cambridge, Lord Heyworth, ex-Chairman Unilever Ltd., and The Hon. Mrs. D. Layton. The Institute developed from the Tavistock Clinic founded in the 1920's.

During the second world war a substantial section of the staff of the Clinic was drawn into the War Office, initially to advise upon the selection and training of officers. They were in fact responsible for the concept and development of the War Office Selection Boards. After the war their expertise was called upon by industry especially in problems which involved the relationship between the individual psychology and the social stresses of the working group. In particular a distinguished series of studies was made at the Glacier Metal Factory Cricklewood, analysing psychological conditions of work and its organisation. The Human Factors Panel of the Lord President's Office (from which the present Human Sciences Division of DSIR has developed) commissioned the Tavistock Institute to do much work on industrial problems. In addition they have been employed almost permanently by Unilever, as consultants upon recruitment and selection of management and the development of new institutions within management. In recent years they have been closely involved in studies of labour turnover, accidents and absenteeism in a variety of industries. As will be seen from Dr. Higgin's biographical notes below, they have done a good deal of work in the Coal Industry under DSIR's auspices. One of their main current projects is as consultants to the Norwegian equivalents of the TUC and FBI, studying "Industrial democracy" in a variety of industries. Their last annual report refers, inter alia, to projects studying decision-making processes in the planning and construction of a steel works; the relationships between petrol retailers and an oil company; and the social and psychological problems of automation.

The Operational Research Society is the professional institute for operational research. It provides a library and information service, arranges technical meetings and publishes abstracts. The techniques of operational research are, of course, now widely used throughout industry and Government.

The Councils of both Institutes have agreed in principle to form an operational research division within the Tavistock Institute. The impetus for this came from the increasing realisation on the part of Tavistock staff that the problems they became involved in often required the analysis of technical processes in operational research terms; and from the realisation in operational research circles that to leave out of their technical studies the social and psychological problems of the working group often left their problems only half solved. (See footnote - p. 85)

Gurth Higgin, M.A., Dip. Ed., Ph. D.

Dr. Higgin is a New Zealander who graduated in Psychology and Education from Victoria University, Wellington. He came to London in 1948 and obtained a Ph.D. (Sociology) at the London School of

Economics. After several years as a sociologist in the Scientific Adviser's Department of the Air Ministry, working on selection, training and morale in the Royal Air Force, he joined the Tavistock Institute in 1954. Since joining the Institute he has been engaged on a long-term research in coal mining and is co-author of a book to be published in 1963 which reports this work. The main purpose of this study was to investigate the interaction of technical change in work at the coal face on the traditional working groups and management structure of underground mining. He has also been involved in other organisational studies, most recently in the field of petroleum distribution, and has published a study of communications in the National Farmers' Union.

Neil Jessop B.Sc., A.R.C.S.

Mr. Jessop is an honours graduate in Mathematics from Imperial College, London, and subsequently specialised in statistics. He has worked as a research statistician in the steel industry and is at present head of operational research in a major industrial company. He is a Fellow of the Royal Statistical Society, a former member of its Council, and he was Vice-President of the Society in 1959. He is the author of numerous papers on operational research and statistics. He is the director designate of the new Institute for Operational Research (Tavistock Institute).

Attachment 2.

EXTRACT FROM A FIRST APPRECIATION OF A RESEARCH PROJECT AND PILOT STUDY ON COMMUNICATIONS FOR THE NATIONAL JOINT CONSULTATIVE COMMITTEE

The Building Process

We have taken as our starting point of the building process a client's building need. The end of the process we have taken as the satisfaction of this client need. At the beginning point of this process the means of achieving the result are in an array of dispersed resources which may be scattered throughout the country. At this point the client is certainly unaware of what resources he needs to achieve his end, and is probably also unaware, except in the broadest terms, of the nature of the construction he requires.

For the present purposes this array of dispersed resources can be thought of as being of two main kinds, technical and social. Here the social aspects of the resources include all the technical, planning, administrative and operational skills and knowledge which people have and which are necessary for the building process.

The technical resources are the materials and equipment that need to be brought together in the appropriate quantities, qualities and at the appropriate times so that they can jointly constitute a finished construction. These may be anywhere, even outside this country.

The approach to these technical resources is through a variety of resource controllers, people and organisations of various kinds whose social resources of knowledge and skill are the means of mobilising the technical resources. These resource controllers, although all independent persons or organisations, depend upon co-operation with others for their activities as none (except in rare instances of large contractors and some public authorities) deploys all the resources called for. A first task, therefore, in the building process is the development from these relationships of interdependent autonomy of a team which is the primary tool of the building process. It is the conjunction in this team of the technical and social resources which allows the operations of the building process to go forward.

Communications of many kinds constitute the energising and controlling factor in the development of the building team. It is through communications that it is conceived, developed and directed in the service of the building process.

The complex patterns of communications which develop are initiated by an approach by the client to a resource controller. This resource controller in turn communicates with others in the name of the client. This initiating function thus puts him in the role of a sponsor of the developing building team. A network of communications is rapidly built up and it is this network which manifests the relationships of the building team and so can be seen to constitute its structure.

All these communications are operations, i.e. activities undertaken to achieve a desired result. These operations in their turn have both a technical and a social aspect. In their techncial aspect they are concerned with the direction and control of a vast range of activities to do with the manipulation and costing of material and equipment. In their social aspect all communications in the building team have some function in the development and maintenance of the network of relationships that constitute the team structure - even the presence or absence of particular people in the distribution of a document is a communication about relationships.

Some forms of formal communication, for example sketch designs, bills of quantities, schedules of components, usually have a much higher technical than social meaning. Others, for example contracts, letters of agreement and most verbal communications, have a higher social content, i.e. have more to do with how people or units relate to each other. But all communications operations contain both aspects in some degree.

Communications Research

The sorts of questions which would need to be asked about the technical aspects of communications would be, for example, what information is being passed by means of this drawing, by this bill of quantities, by this specification, and why is it in this form? Is there another, perhaps completely different, way of passing this information? How do key people in the building team receive the information they need and how do they transmit information to others? Do they get sufficient information at the appropriate time? Do they get more than they need, or not enough, and if so, why? Are all the technical resources (including money) being employed appropriate as to quality, quantity and timing for the job in hand, and are all those that are appropriate being employed? Is there a comprehensive plan to provide a yardstick for all these sorts of question, e.g. a Critical Path Analysis? And inevitably in such enquiries there will be the intrusion of the question of how and to what extent the social function of communi cations is interfering with or assisting their technical function.

As the social aspects of the communications operations embody the fabric of the building team structure it would be necessary in the first phase of the research to learn something of the way in which the teams get built up from among interdependent autonomous units. Is 'team', with its overtones of esprit de corps and a shared goal, the correct term? What is the sponsor role? How is this role handled by the architect, the man who usually takes it? Is it handled differently if it is taken by some other resource controller? What are the implications of an internal sponsorship role (as with some big firms and most local authorities)? In a building team are there other similar sponsor roles, e.g. a contractor vis-a-vis sub-contractors? Are there, among the variety of size and of resource-mix involved in teams for different building processes, recognisable types? If so, can these be identified and by what characteristics, and do they have different qualities of relationship and communication? What type of team is best for what type of job?

More generally it would be necessary to know something about the traditional, personal, commercial or other reasons why the relationships among the various types of building team are what they are. It is in the communications between these units that these relationships are created and maintained and where the mutual help, hindrances, rivalries, likes and dislikes express themselves overtly and covertly. Something of all this would need to be known so that the effect on the building process of these different patterns of relationships could be seen,and other models designed to improve the relationships and hence the communications.

Tavistock Institute
August 1962

APPENDIX B

THE BUILDING TEAM RATING SCALE

1. As recorded in the body of the report, quite early in our a acquaintance with the industry we formed the impression that there is a fairly widespread confusion about definitions of the roles of the many occupations involved in the building process. There seemed to be no clear and commonly-held understandings of just what sort of people are in different roles and what they actually do, or could normally be expected to do. For any role it always seemed to come down to a question of "it all depends".

2. If this impression was correct it had obvious implications for further study of relationships and communications in the building team, and as our contacts were necessarily limited a means of making some sort of test of it was obviously essential. On the grounds that any evidence is better than none, we devised the attached questionnaire and covering letter to take a first very rough sounding.

3. When there is a work situation, as in the building industry, calling for a "division of labour" of one overall job into many different levels of skill, if the situation is fairly stable everybody in all the different roles involved has a very similar understanding of what everybody else does, i.e. of the nature of their contribution to the whole job. Moreover, in such a stable situation the different occupations associated with the different roles develop a commonly understood general standing in terms of the whole of society, i.e. they develop a known social status. Consider the roles in a hospital, for example. There are porters, housemen, nurses, registrars, technicians, ward maids, consultants, and so on. All have a fairly clear idea of what everybody else contributes to the work of the hospital and what the social status is of each of the different occupations involved. Our impression was that this sort of stability did not hold for the building industry. Hence the questions on our questionnaire.

The Results

4. We sent out some 220 forms to a sample covering all the occupations mentioned in the questionnaire. To date (beginning of March) we have had 119 completed forms returned. Some have come in since the time when tabulation had to be started, so results are presented for only 97.

5. Many respondents found the questions difficult to answer and somewhat annoying, and it was clear that they would have liked to expand and qualify their ratings so as to do justice to their knowledge of the roles played by the various occupations in the building process. There is also the complication of the different interpretations put on the titles of the roles. For these reasons and because the sample is small, and in particular because of the small size of some of the sub-samples, the material is treated only by simple tabulation and no statistical procedures have been applied. The results must therefore be regarded as tentative and of corroborative value only.

6. Replies were received from nine clients, fourteen architects, fifteen quantity surveyors, nine consulting engineers specialising in structural and civil engineering, one consultant engineer specialising in services, thirteen builders and civil engineering contractors, seven general builders (the difference between the building contractor and the general builder being defined largely in terms of size and type of building constructed (11)) fifteen sub-contractors, seven manufacturer/suppliers and nine builders' merchants. No replies were received from sub-traders.

7. Nine replies had to be excluded because they did not indicate the respondent's own occupation. Sub-samples with fewer than seven respondents were excluded from the analysis. Thus no analysis could be made of the way sub-traders and consulting engineers specialising in services rated the other occupations, though there is of course material on how these two occupations were rated by the others.

8. The first support we had for our impression of instability came from the many letters we received. Some said the roles were too confused to be able to make any meaningful ratings, and did not attempt to do so. Many others who did attempt the exercise added qualifications, of which the comment that 'In both columns the evaluations will vary widely from one job to another" is very typical.

9. Figure 1 shows the average (mean) ratings by the whole sample for each occupation. In each case the top shaded bar represents the average rating of the occupation for its "contribution to the building process", and the lower unshaded bar represents its average rating for "social status". In the case of clients no rating of social status was asked for because it was thought that this would vary too much for

anyone to be able to make a general statement about it.

10. In the analyses that follow these averages, given by the whole sample of 97, are used as the only base line available for observing the extent of variations in the perceptions of all the occupations of themselves and of each other. The averages must not, of course, be thought of as necessarily "true" measures of contribution or social status. A much wider survey and analysis would be required to establish measures of that kind. Here we are concerned only with the extent of variation in the perceptions of different groups of the same phenomena.

11. It will be seen from figures 2 to 12 that there is a very wide range of variation in the ratings assigned to each occupation, especially the ratings on contribution to the building process. The status ratings are less variable. It must be remembered that these are variations between the averages for the various occupations doing the rating. Variation within the total sample treated as individuals would be much greater.

12. The range of variation is greatest on clients, where there is a difference of 41 points between the lowest and the highest scores. This is two-fifths of the total scale from 0 to 100. This wide variation on clients is hardly surprising, however, since there are many different types of client, and the people doing the rating may have had different types of experience with clients.

13. The lowest range of variation is found for builders and civil engineering contractors (15 points). On the other occupations there is a variation of 20 to 24 points, representing one-fifth to one quarter of the total scale. These are the figures when self-ratings are left out. If self-ratings are included the range of variation is very much higher.

14. Unfortunately there are no comparable data from other similar situations of known stability or instability to put against these observed variations among building occupations. Nevertheless, these results do suggest a situation of instability lacking very clearly defined and widely agreed views of the roles of the different occupations in the building process. In this they are in keeping with our field impression, and so give corroboration to it.

Ratings Made by Each Occupation

15. Figures 13 to 21 show the same material from a different point of

view. Instead of showing the average ratings given to each occupation as in figures 2 to 12, figures 13 to 21 show the average ratings given by each occupation. In each case "contribution to the building process" and "social status" ratings are shown together, and the average on each for the whole sample is also shown. If there is a difference of more than five points between an average rating by a particular occupation and the corresponding average given by the total sample, it is probably worthy of note.

16. It is tempting to explore the implications of these figures further to see if one's impressions of the nature of the relationships between different groups is borne out. Of particular interest is a matching of the ratings given to each other by particular pairs. As the numbers in the sample are so small and the method of its selection so haphazard, however, we do not feel justified in reporting such detailed analysis.

COVERING LETTER SENT WITH THE QUESTIONNAIRE

I am at present engaged on a pilot study of communications in the building industry in conjunction with members of the Operational Research Society on behalf of the National Joint Consultative Committee.

My Operational Research colleagues are developing a model of the building process which we hope will lead to practical suggestions about improving methods of communication. My function as a sociologist is to find out something of the social relationships and attitudes among those involved in the building operation. From this some idea of the social climate in the industry can be known and the sorts of attitudes and beliefs about others that would help or hinder the development of better communications can be understood in a way that will allow fruitful examination and discussion of them by all concerned.

To help me in this job I have drawn up a simple questionnaire, a copy of which I enclose. You will appreciate that it is only by having a large and widely representative number of these forms returned that it becomes of use. I would be very grateful therefore if you would be good enough to complete it and return it to me anonymously.

Thank you.

Yours sincerely,

(Dr. G.W. Higgin)

CONFIDENTIAL TO DR. G. HIGGIN - TAVISTOCK INSTITUTE

BUILDING TEAM RATING SCALES

Would you indicate on a scale from 0 to 100 the ratings you would give the following members of the building team on scales of social status and of the importance of their contribution to the whole building process from conception to completion.

Please give your opinion of the typical rather than the ideal rating in each case, and use your own every-day definition of social status and importance of contribution.

Would you first decide whom you rate highest and give that role 100, then rate the others in relation to this. Equal ratings (even at 100) are of course possible and, if you wish, minus ratings. The ratings in one column do not, of course, add up to 100.

Would you indicate below which is your own role among those mentioned.

If you wish to add any comments please feel free to do so.

	Social Status	Contribution to the Building Process
Architect	....	....
Builder and Civil Engineer Contractor	....	....
Builders' Merchant	....	....
Consulting Engineer		
(a) Structural and Civil	....	....
(b) Services	....	....
General Builder	....	....
Manufacturer/Supplier (including plant)	....	....
Quantity Surveyor	....	....
Sub-Contractor	....	....
Sub-Trader (Plasterer, plumber, etc.)	....	....
Client	N.A.	....

My own role is: ....

Comments:

FIGURE 1: Average Ratings by the Whole Sample of 'Contribution to the Building Process' and 'Social Status' for Each Occupation.

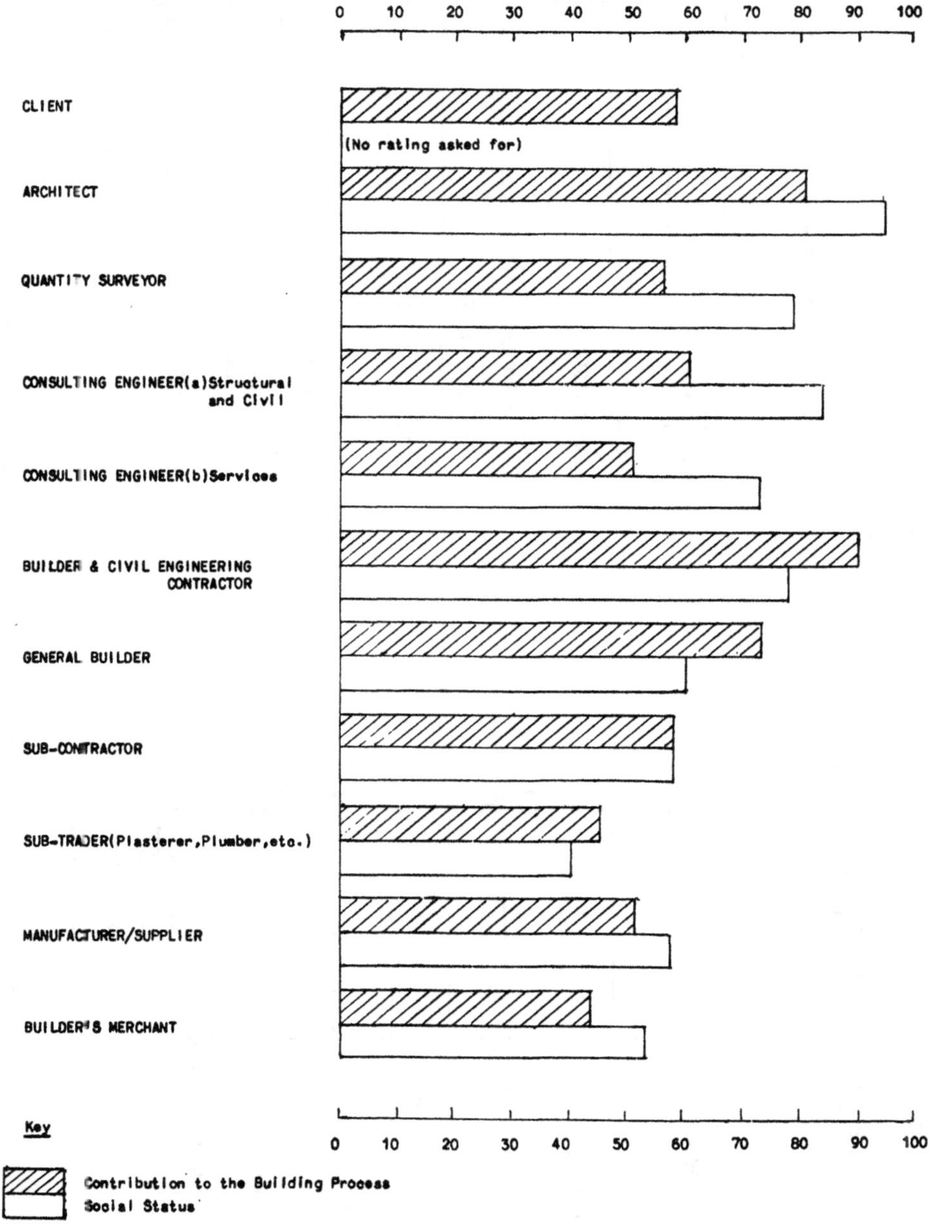

G

FIGURE 3: The Occupation of ARCHITECT as rated for 'Contribution to the Building Process'

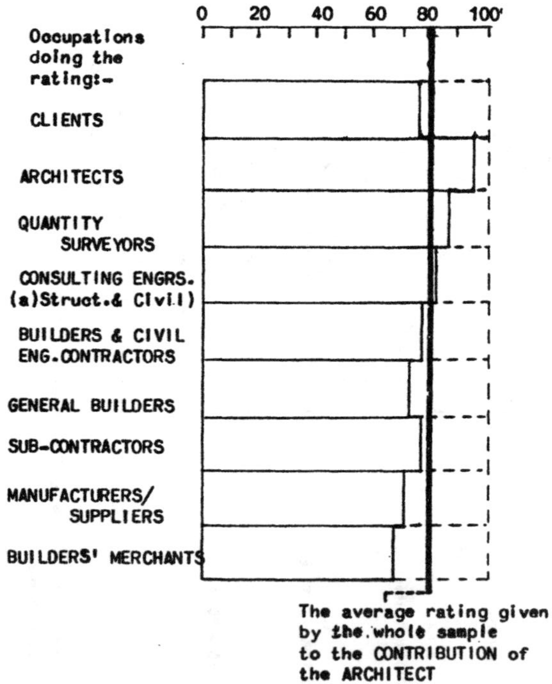

The Occupation of ARCHITECT as rated for 'Social Status'

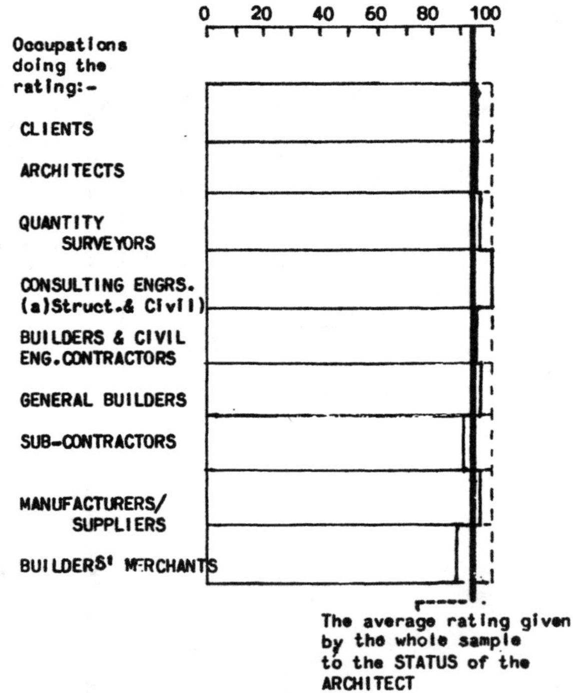

FIGURE 2: The role of CLIENT as rated for 'Contribution to the Building Process'

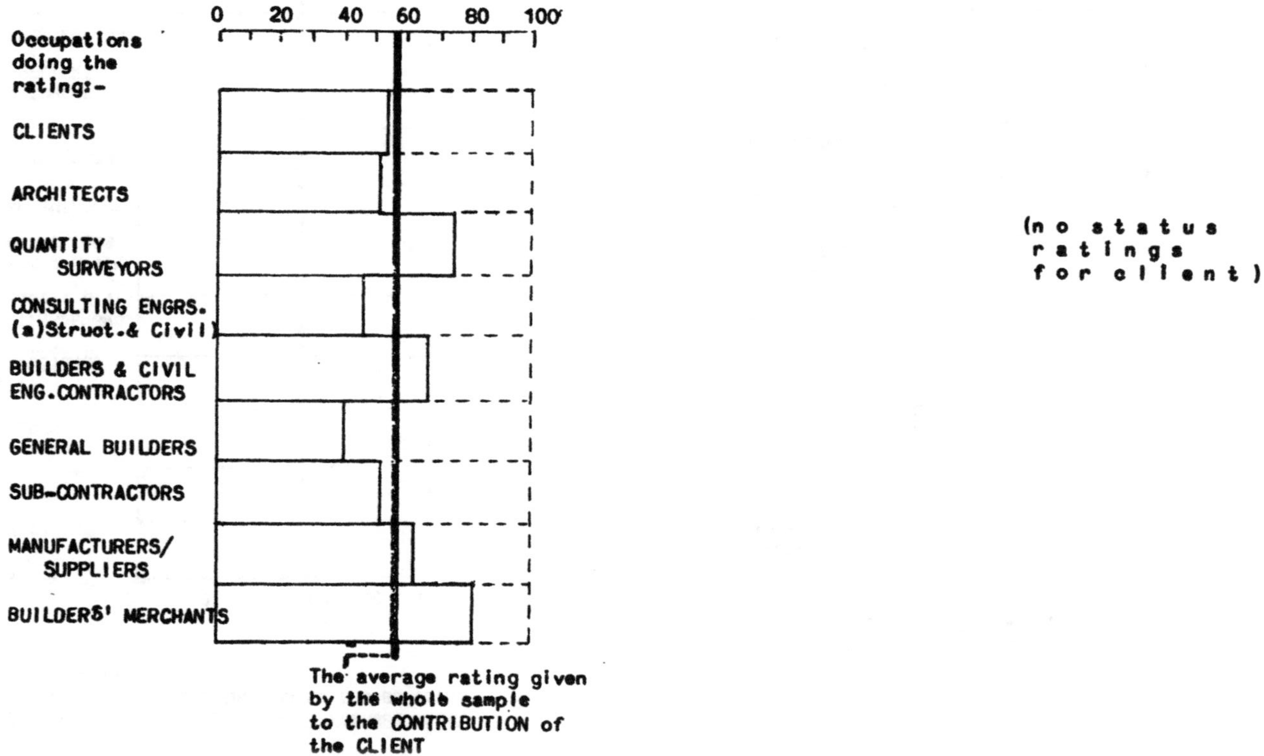

FIGURE 4: The Occupation of QUANTITY SURVEYOR as rated for 'Contribution to the Building Process'

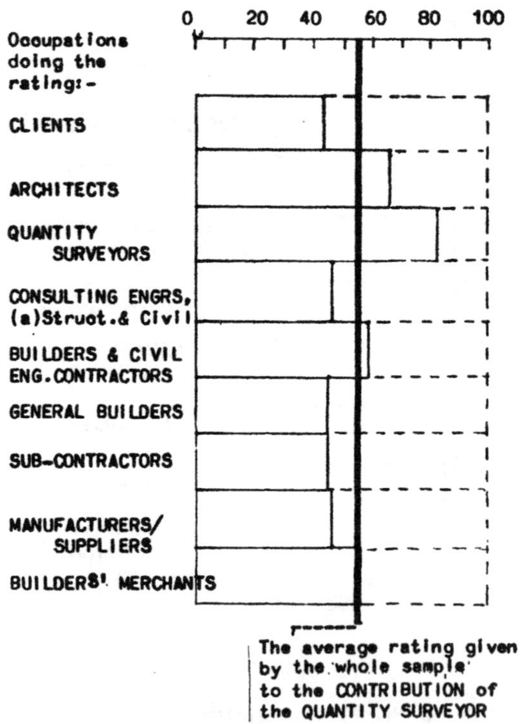

The Occupation of QUANTITY SURVEYOR as rated for 'Social Status'

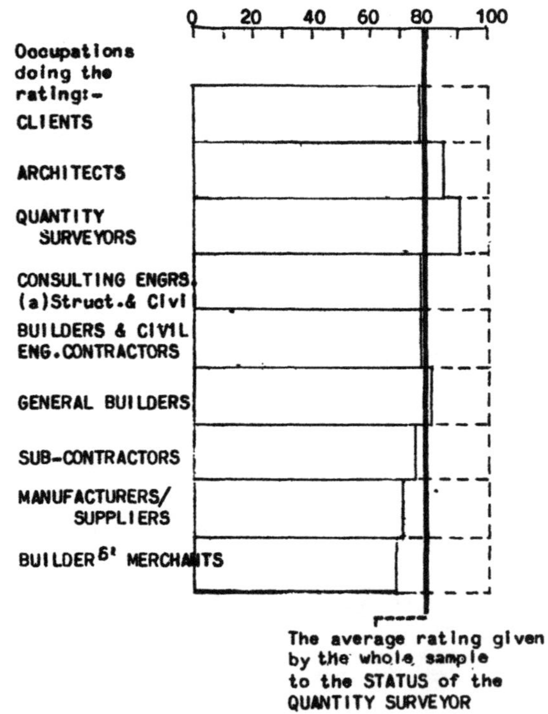

FIGURE 5: The Occupation of CONSULTING ENGINEER (Structural & Civil) as rated for-'Contribution to the Building Process'

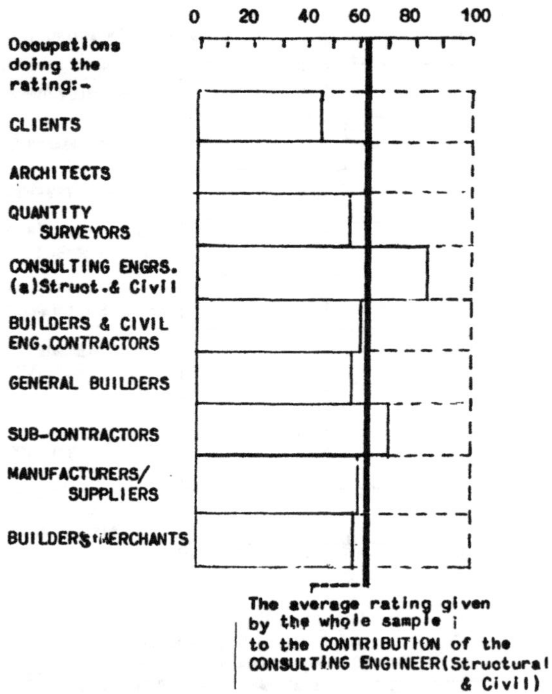

The Occupation of CONSULTING ENGINEER (Structural & Civil) as rated for 'Social Status

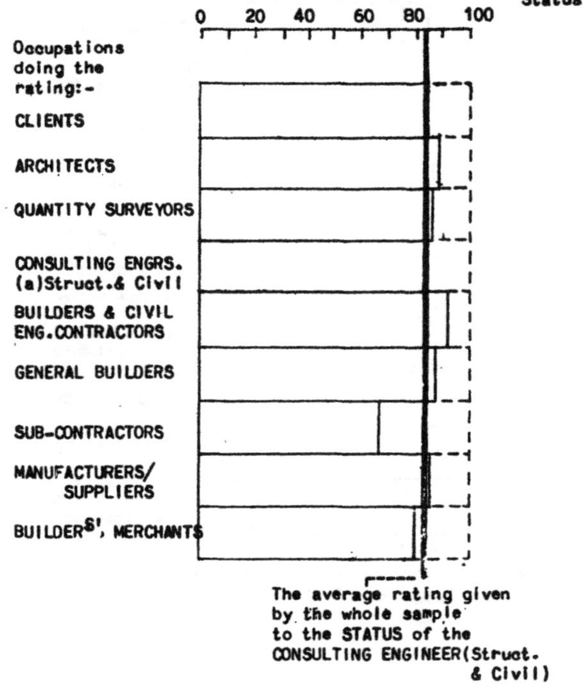

FIGURE 6: The Occupation of CONSULTING ENGINEER (Services) as rated for 'Contribution to the Building Process'

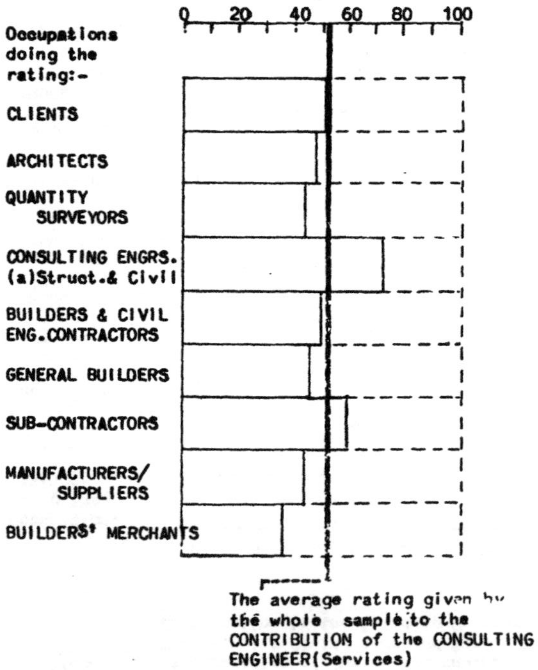

The Occupation of CONSULTING ENGINEER (Services) as rated for 'Social Status'

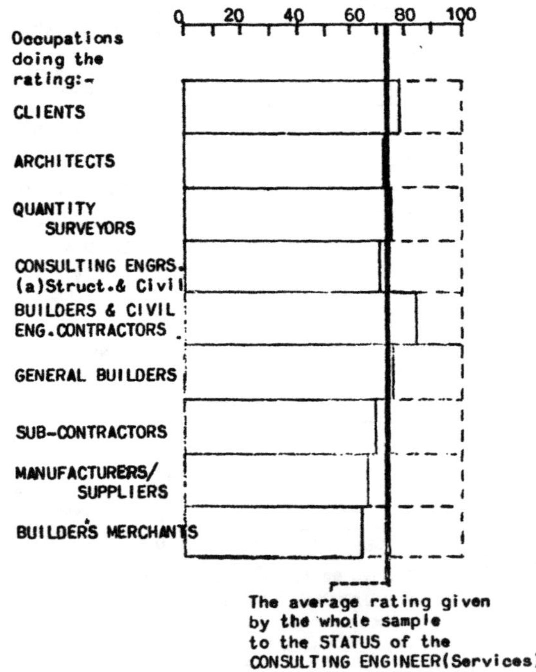

FIGURE 7: The Occupation of BUILDER AND CIVIL ENGINEERING CONTRACTOR as rated for- 'Contribution to the Building Process'

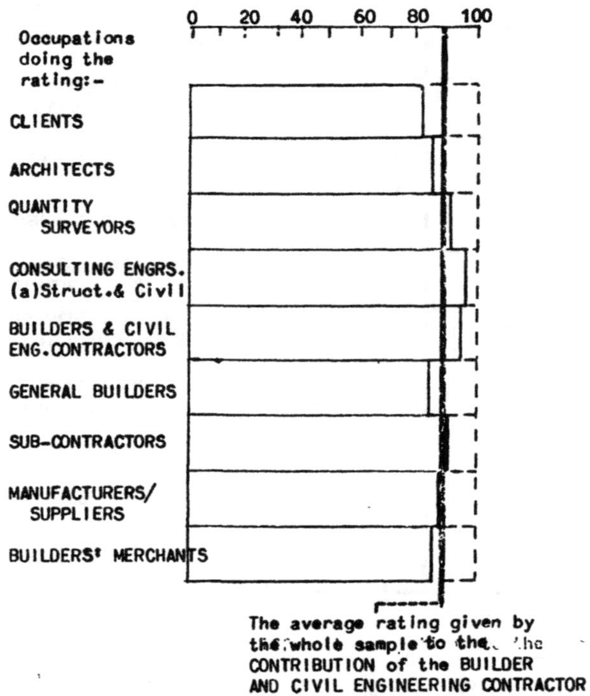

The Occupation of BUILDER AND CIVIL ENG. CONTRACTOR as rated for- 'Social Status'

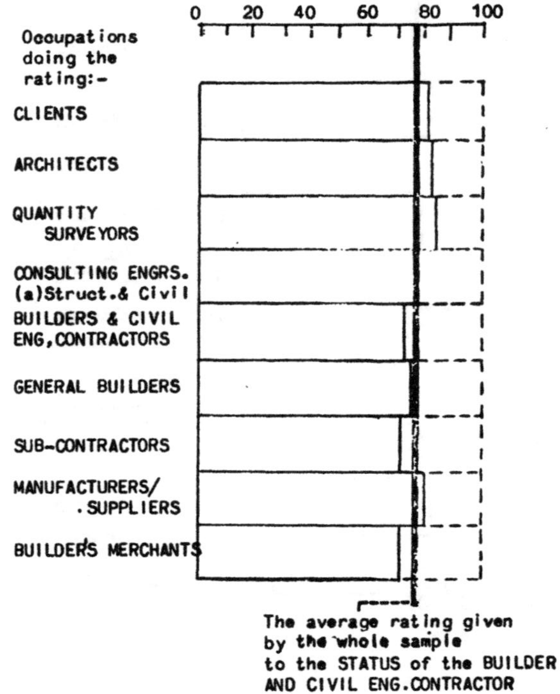

FIGURE 8: The Occupation of GENERAL BUILDER as rated for – 'Contribution to the Building Process'

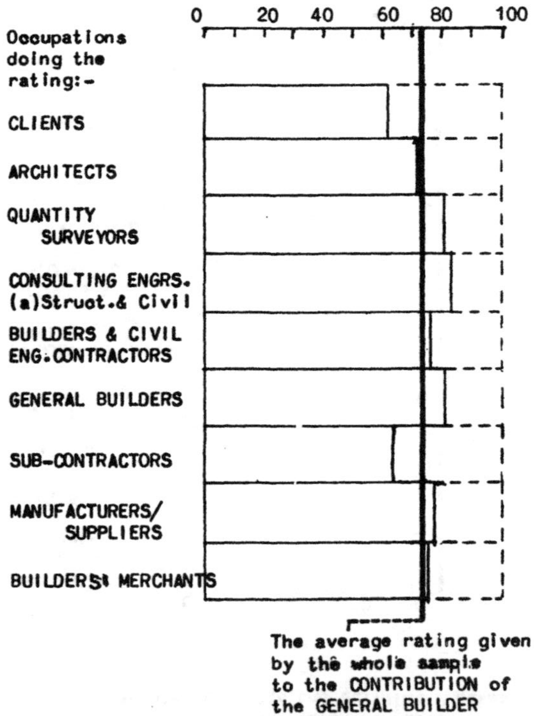

The Occupation of GENERAL BUILDER as rated 'for-'Social Status'

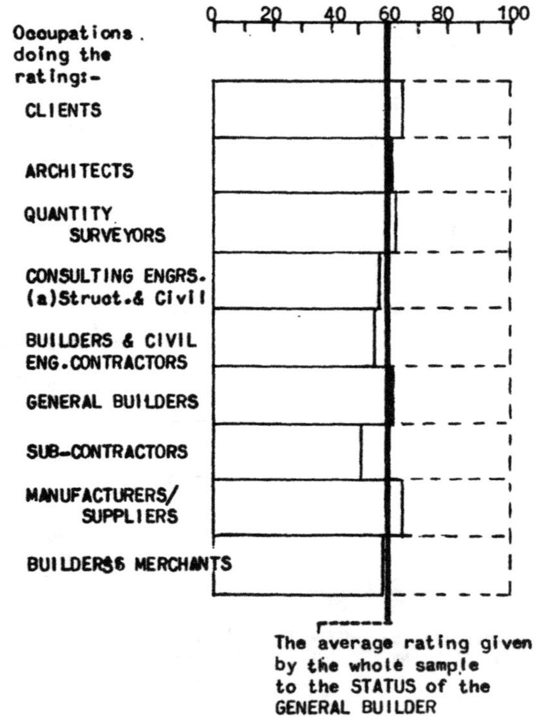

FIGURE 9: The Occupation of SUB-CONTRACTOR as rated for – 'Contribution to the Building Process'

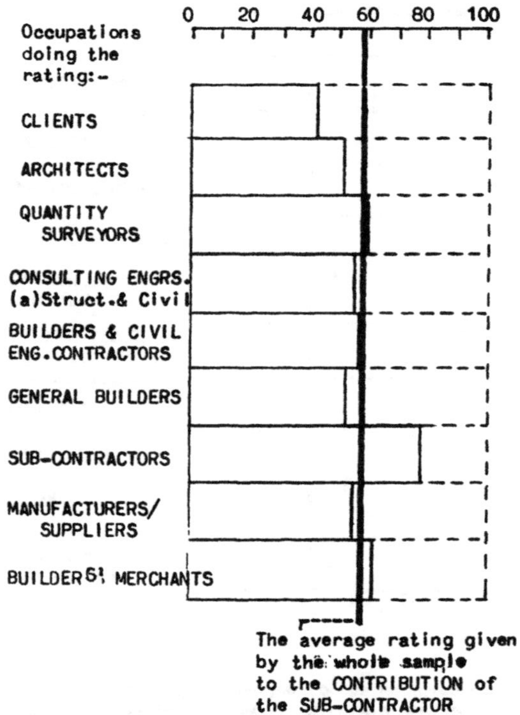

The Occupation of SUB-CONTRACTOR as rated for – 'Social Status'

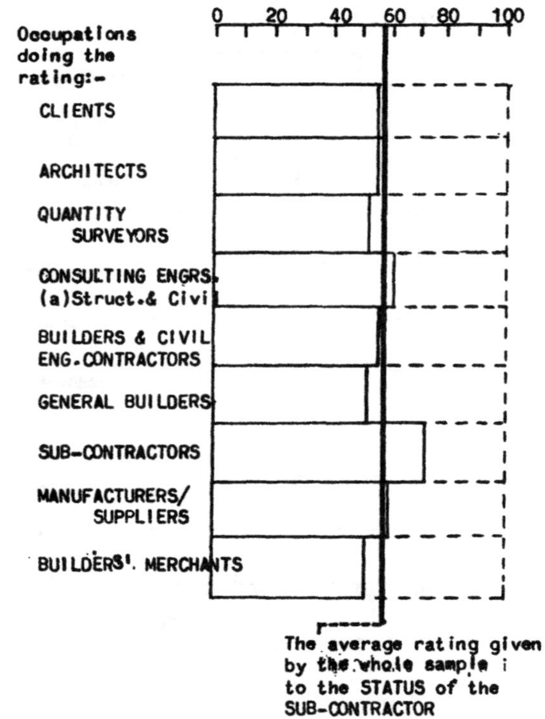

FIGURE 12: The Occupation of BUILDER'S MERCHANT as rated for – 'Contribution to the Building Process'

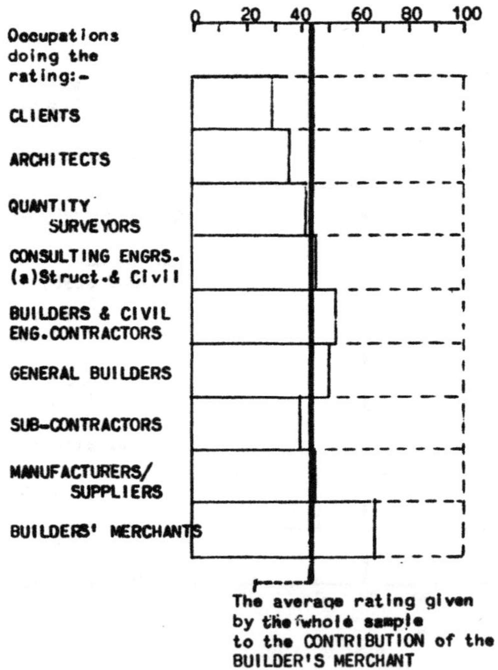

The Occupation of BUILDER'S MERCHANT as rated for – 'Social Status'

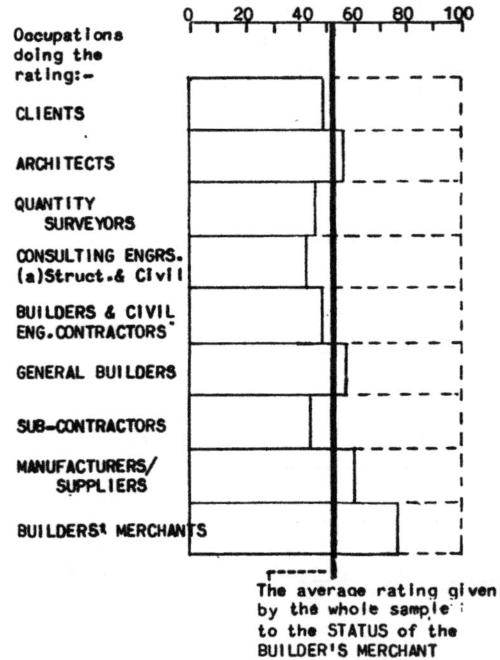

FIGURE 13: The Average Ratings given to Each Occupation by - CLIENTS

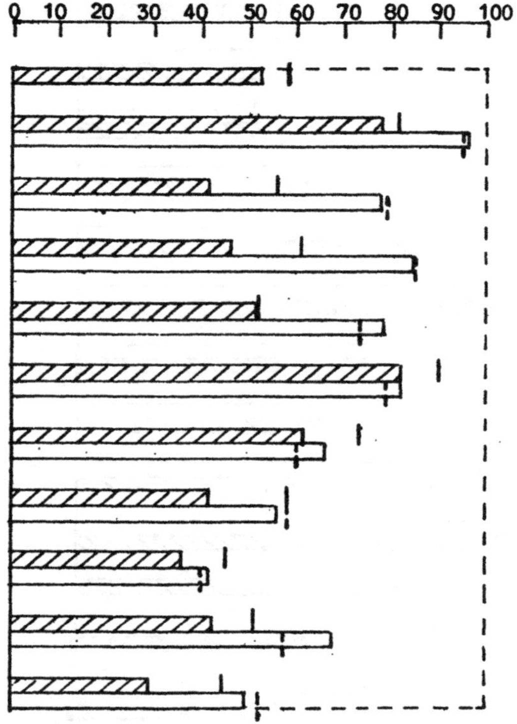

Occupations being rated

CLIENT

ARCHITECT

QUANTITY SURVEYOR

CONSULTING ENGINEER (a) Struct. & Civil

CONSULTING ENGINEER (b) Services

BUILDER AND CIVIL ENG. CONTRACTOR

GENERAL BUILDER

SUB-CONTRACTOR

SUB-TRADER

MANUFACTURER/SUPPLIER

BUILDER'S MERCHANT

FIGURE 14: The Average Ratings given to Each Occupation by - ARCHITECTS

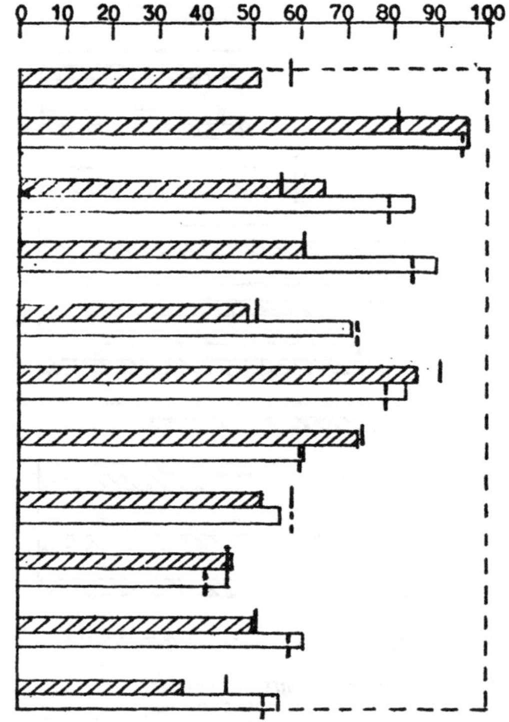

FIGURE 15: The Average Ratings given to Each Occupation by - QUANTITY SURVEYORS

FIGURE 16: The Average Ratings given to Each Occupation by - CONSULTING ENGINEERS(a)Structural and Civil

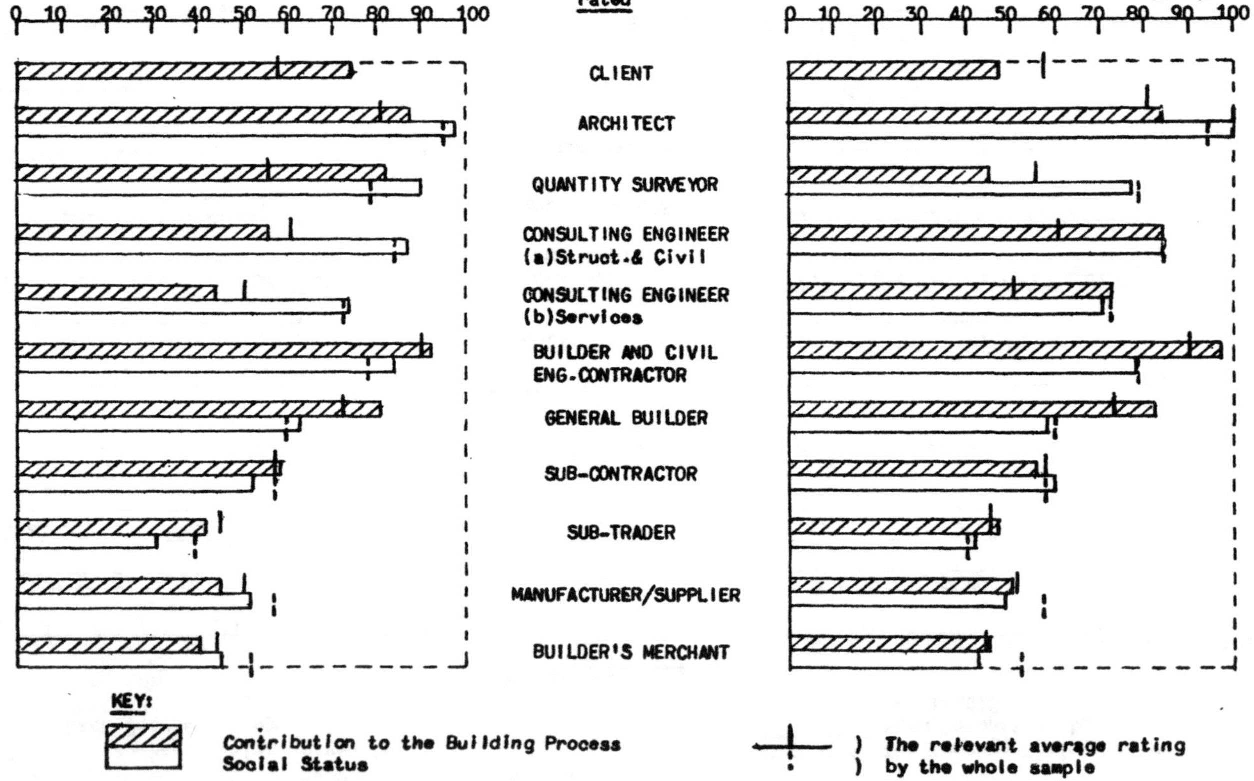

FIGURE 17: The Average Ratings given to Each Occupation by - BUILDERS & CIVIL ENG. CONTRACTORS

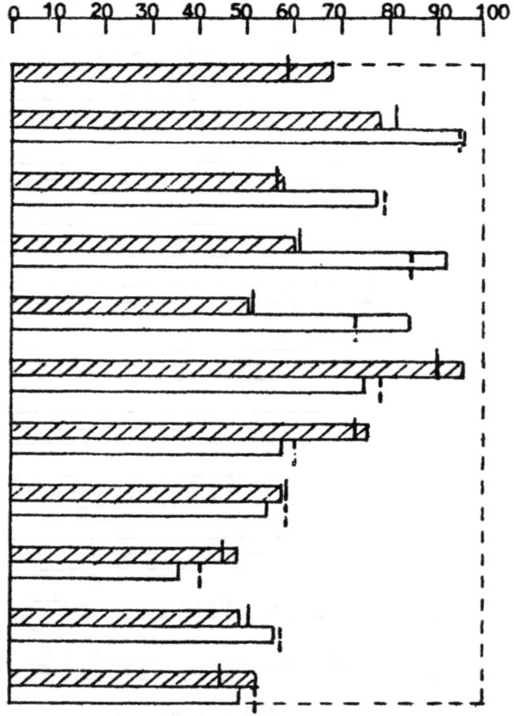

Occupations being rated

CLIENT

ARCHITECT

QUANTITY SURVEYOR

CONSULTING ENGINEER (a)Struct. & Civil

CONSULTING ENGINEER (b)Services

BUILDER AND CIVIL ENG. CONTRACTOR

GENERAL BUILDER

SUB-CONTRACTOR

SUB-TRADER

MANUFACTURER/SUPPLIER

BUILDER'S MERCHANT

FIGURE 18: The Average Ratings given to Each Occupation by - GENERAL BUILDERS

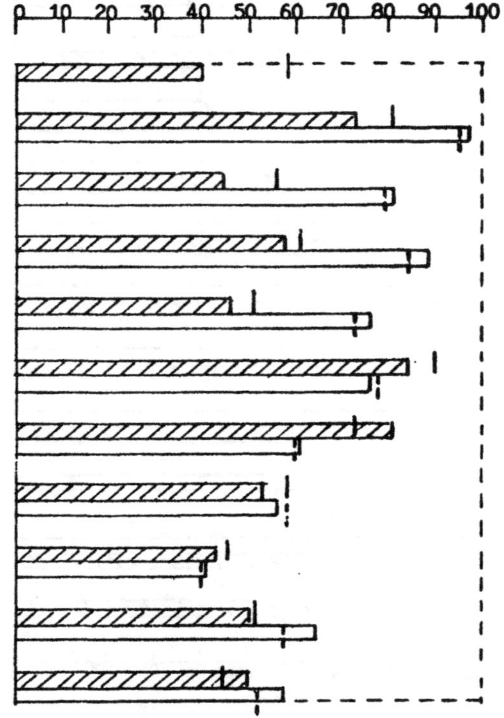

FIGURE 19: The Average Ratings given to Each Occupation by - SUB-CONTRACTORS

FIGURE 20: The Average Ratings given to Each Occupation by - MANUFACTURER/SUPPLIERS

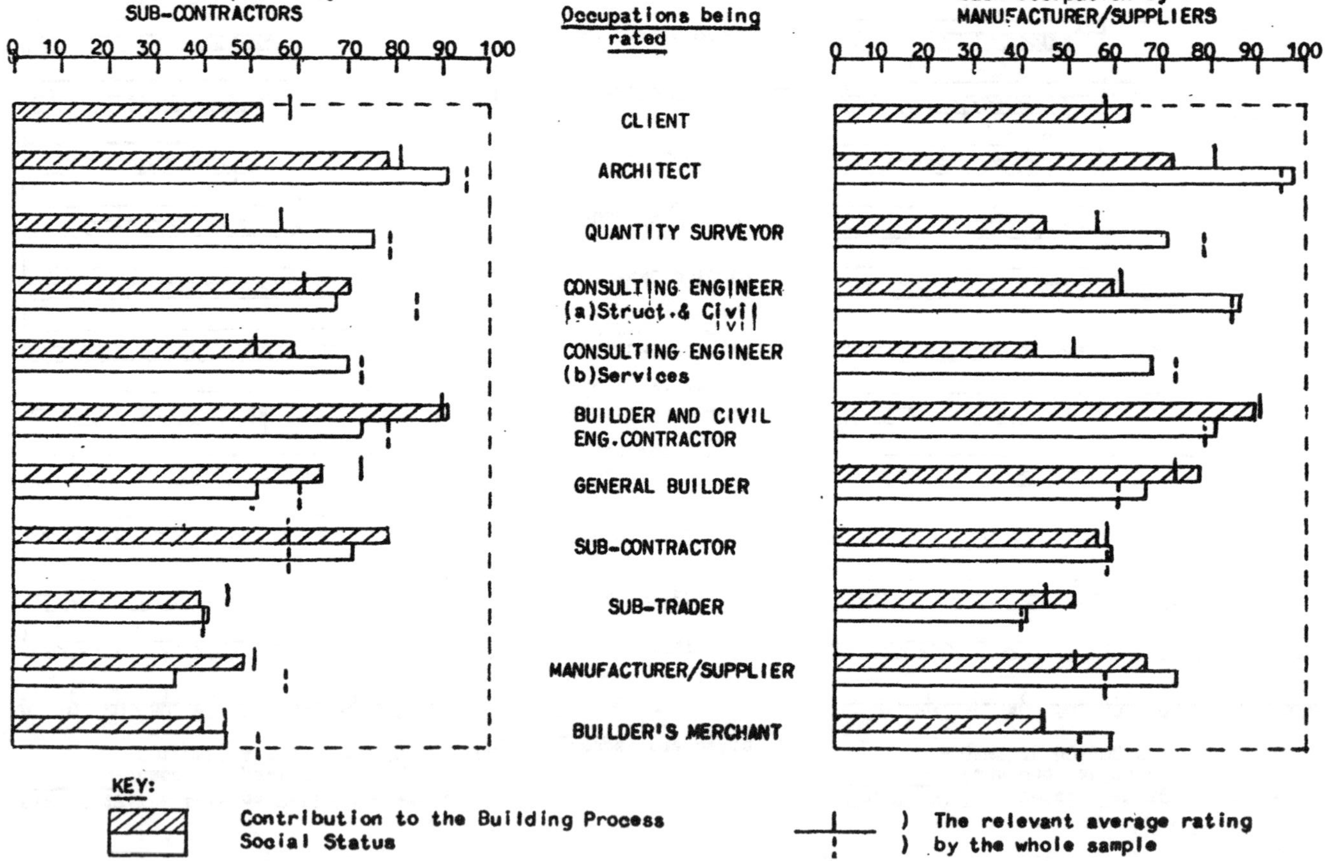

FIGURE 21: The Average Ratings given to Each Occupation by - BUILDERS' MERCHANTS

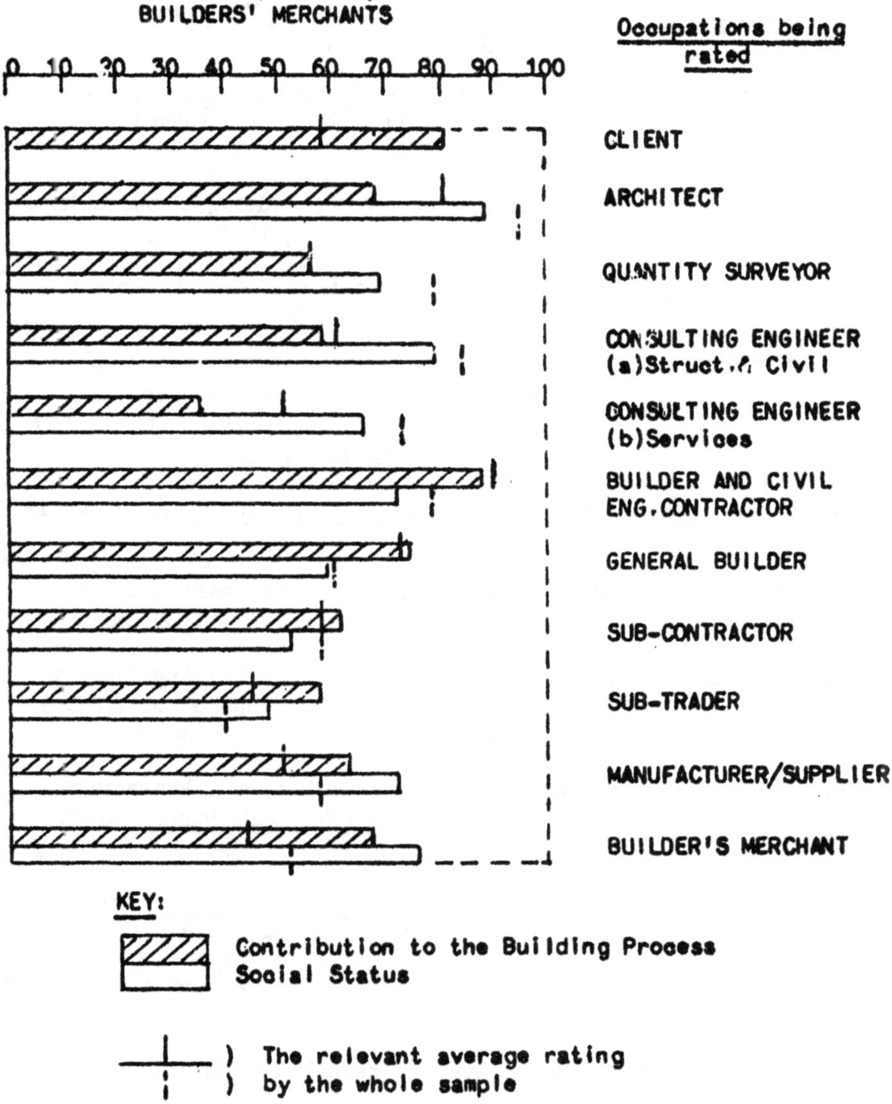

REFERENCES

1. A-Group, Pilot Architectural Documents for Designing, Stockholm, June, 1961.

2. ALBERT, Kenneth, Policy for the Building Industry, Fabian Research Series, No. 170, London Fabian Society, 1955.

3. Anglo-American Council on Productivity, Building. Productivity Team Report, London, 1950.

4. Aqua Group (The), Pre-contract Practice, Crosby Lockwood & Son Ltd., London, 1960.

5. BENNET, Sir Thomas and WOODBINE PARISH, D.E. The Organisation of the Building Industry and the Architect's Responsibilities, J. R.I.B.A. Vol. 62, No. 8, June 1955.

6. B.I.M. Management Training in the Building Industry, London 1956.

7. BISHOP, D., 'Mechanisation and Building Processes', Structural Concrete, March/April 1 (2) 1962.

8. BLASHILL, T., The Present Condition of the Building Industry A paper and discussion reported in R.I.C.S. Transactions Vol. XXXIII (1900-01)

9. BOWEN, I. and ELLIS, A.W.T. The Building and Contracting Industry, Oxford Economic Papers No. 7, March 1945.

10. British Productivity Council, A Review of Productivity in the Building Industry, London, undated.

11. Builder (The) The Building Industry ... 1962 onward, London, 1962.

12. CANNELL, J.B. 'A New System Needed', The Builder, Vol. CXCVI, No. 6054, April 1959.

13. CARTER, C.F. The Building Industry, The Structure of British Industry Vol. 1, C.U.P. 1958.

14. Central Council for Works and Buildings, The Planning and Management of Building Contracts (Simon report), H.M.S.O. London, 1944.

15. Contract Journal, Planning and Management of Contracts, August 1962.

16. DALE, K.K. Future Practice and Procedure in Quantity Surveying, A paper and discussion reported in The Chartered Surveyor, Vol 93, Nos. 6 & 7, Dec. 1960 & Jan. 1961.

17. D.S.I.R. Incentives in Building, London, 1959

18. EMMERSON, Sir Harold Survey of Problems before the Construction Industries, H.M.S.O. London, 1962.

19. Financial Times (The), The Analytic Approach to Work, (Network Analysis in Building) and correspondence following, 11th and 20th February, 1963.

20. GRAFTON, P.W., Building - The Emerging Pattern, The Builder, No. 6238, 7th December, 1962.

21. GREEN, Robert, The Architect's Guide to Running a Job, The Architectural Press, London, 1962.

22. Guardian (The), The Builder goes Bankrupt. Bill to protect public. 27th February 1963.

23. Guardian (The), 'Communion' The Report of the building of a Church, 6th December, 1962.

24. Guardian (The), 'The Package Deal', and correspondence following 28th January, 1st/14th/18th/20th February, 1963.

25. Institute of Builders (The), Management Studies for the Building Industry, London, 1959.

26. JONES, I.E., Building by Direct Labour, Federated Employers Press, London, undated.

27. KNIGHT, T.L., Economics of Multi-storey Flats Construction, Keystone, Vol. 32, No. 4, 1957

28. LAYTON, Elizabeth, Building by Local Authorities, George Allen & Unwin, London, 1961.

29. LAYTON, Elizabeth, The Practical Training of Architects, R.I.B.A. London, 1962.

30. LEA, F.M., The Building Industry in an Expanding Economy, J. R.I.B.A., Vol. 69, No. 7, July 1962.

31. LEE, Michael, The Evolution of the Bill of Quantities. A paper for the working party on quantity surveying techniques, Q.S. Committee, R.I.C.S., 1963.

32. L.M.B.A., 'Tomorrow's Builder', London, undated.

33. L.M.B.A. and F.A.S.S., 'Co-operation between Main Contractors and Sub-contractors in the Building Industry', Report of a Joint Conference, March 1961.

34. L.M.B.A. and N.J.C.C., 'Communications in the Building Industry' Report of a Conference at Sundridge Park Management Centre, November 1958.

35. Ministry of Education, Notes on the CLASP System of Construction for the 12th Milan Triennale.

36. Ministry of Education, Pamphlet No. 4 'Building Crafts', H.M.S.O. London, 1945.

37. Monopolies and Restrictive Practices Commission, Report on the Supply of Buildings in the Greater London Area, 1954. H.M.S.O. London.

38. N.F.B.P.M. The Distribution of Building Materials, London, undated.

39. N.F.B.T.E., Accounting Methods for the Small Builder, London undated.

40. N.F.B.T.O., The N.F.B.T.O. and the 40-hour week, Memo. February, 1963.

41. N.J.C.C., A Code of Procedure for Selective Tendering, London, 1959.

42. N.J.C.C., Proceedings of Annual Conferences of Regional Chairmen and Secretaries, 1961 and 1962.

43. N.J.C.C., Report of a Joint Committee on Tendering Procedure, (The Howard Robertson Report), London, 1954.

44. National Joint Council for the Building Industry, Report of the National Joint Apprenticeship Board.

45. National Joint Council for the Building Industry, National Working Rules for the Building Industry, London 1960.

46. NISBET, J., Quantity Surveying in London during the Nineteenth Century, Jnl. of the R.I.C.S., Vol. XXXI, Part VIII, February, 1952.

47. NISBET, J., The Role of the Quantity Surveyor during the Design Stage, The Chartered Surveyor, Vol. 92, No. 1, July 1959.

48. NUTTALL, J.F., Some Principles of the Production Control of Building Work, Journal of Industrial Economics, Vol. 10, No. 1, November 1961.

49. POSTGATE, R.W., The Builders' History, N.F.B.T.O., London, 1923.

50. REINERS, W.J., Research, Cost Planning and Cost Control, The National Builder, Vol. 39, No. 9, April 1959.

51. REINERS, W.J. and ALSOP, K., Information for the Building Industry in the United Kingdom, Innovation in Building, Contributions at the 2nd C.I.B. Congress, Cambridge, 1962.

52. R.I.B.A., The Architect and His Office, London, 1962.

53. R.I.B.A., The Architect as Arbitrator, London, 1959.

54. R.I.B.A. and N.F.B.T.E., The Building Owner and Planning in Advance. A Joint Statement, Undated.

55. R.I.C.S., The Chartered Quantity Surveyor and 'Package' Contracts, Memo, dated January 1963.

56. R.I.C.S. Cost Research Panel, Cost Planning, The Chartered Surveyor, Vol. 92, No. 3, September 1959.

57. R.I.C.S. Cost Research Panel, The Function and Uses of the Bill of Quantities, The Chartered Surveyor, Vol. 95, No. 6, December 1962.

58. R.I.C.S. and N.F.B.T.E., Standard Method of Measurement of Building Works, London, 1962.

59. STONE, P.A., Hospital Planning and Decision Techniques, The Hospital, Vol. 58, Part II, November 1962.

60. STONE, P.A. and REINERS, W.J., Organisation and Efficiency of the House-building Industry in England and Wales, Journal of Industrial Economics, Vol. II, April, 1954.

61. Sunday Times (The), A Revolutionary at the Ministry, (M.P.B.W.) March 3rd, 1963.

62. TRENCH, P., Looking Ahead, The National Builder, April 1960.

63. Times (The), Correspondence on The Building Industry, 9th November, 1962.

64. Times (The), Mr. Hare Enters the Maze: Labour Relations at Building Sites, 10th December, 1962.

65. WALTERS, R.T., The Future of Building: The Need for an Investigation into the Changing Structure of the Building Industry, J. R.I.B.A., Vol, 57, No. 7, May, 1950.

66. WALTERS, R.T., The Structure of the Building Industry, J. R.I.B.A., November 1959.

67. WESTON, J.C., Building Management, Technology, Vol. III, No. 3, March 1962.

68. WESTON, J.C., Research into the Interplay of Design and Production, J. R.I.B.A., Vol. 67, No. 4, February 1960.

69. Working Party on Building Operations (Ministry of Works), Report on Building, H.M.S.O., London, 1950.

EPILOGUE

MEMBERS OF THE COMMUNICATIONS RESEARCH COMMITTEE

Lord James of Rusholme (Chairman)	Vice-Chancellor, University of York.
Mr. J.F. Bradford	F. Bradford & Co. Ltd. Ferro-concrete Engineers & Contractors.
Mr. Eric Caswell	Chairman, The Metal Window Association Ltd.
Mr. R. Chapman	President, The National Federation of Builders' & Plumbers' Merchants.
Mr. A.B. Cherns, M.A.	Secretary, Human Sciences Committee, Department of Scientific & Industrial Research
Mr. Andrew Derbyshire	Senior Architect to Messrs. Robert Matthew, Johnson-Marshall & Partners.
Mr. J.B. Dick	Deputy Chief Scientific Officer, Building Research Station.
Mr. Basil Engert	Engert & Rolfe Ltd., Roofing Felt & Asphalt Manufacturers.
Mr. N.S. Farrow, OBE	Howard Farrow Ltd., Civil Engineering & Building Contractors.

Mr. P.W. Grafton	Messrs. G.D. Walford & Partners, Chartered Quantity Surveyors.
Sir William Holford	Professor of Town Planning, University College, London.
Mr. J.P. Inglis	Drake & Gorham Contractors Ltd., Electrical, Mechanical & Hydraulic Engineers.
Mr. J.W.J. Leslie	Messrs. Barlow, Leslie & Partners, Consulting Electrical & Mechanical Engineers.
Mr. Frank Newby	Messrs. Felix J. Samuely & Partners, Consulting Engineers.
Mr. D.E. Woodbine Parish, CBE	Bovis Ltd., Building Contractors.
Mr. E.R. Parrinder	Messrs. Davis, Belfield & Everest, Chartered Quantity Surveyors.
Mr. W.J. Reiners	Director of Research & Information Ministry of Public Building Research & Development, Ministry
Mr. W.H. Shouksmith	J.H. Shouksmith & Son Ltd., Plumbers & Glaziers.
Mr. R.T. Walters	Deputy-Director-General of Research & Development, Ministry of Public Building & Works.
Mr. Harry Weaver	General Secretary, National Federation of Building Trades Operatives.
Mr. A.M. Lewis	Royal Institute of British Architects.

(Secretary to the Board of Trustees and the Communications Research Committee)

When the Communications Research Committee took over responsibility for this research on behalf of the Building Industry as a whole, we found we had two starting points. The first was the general directive we had from the Project Trustees. Their Trust Deed charges them to promote "research into the patterns of operations involved in the building process ... the study of the respective roles of and relationships between the members of the building team... (and) the setting up and testing of research models for improving communications ...". These activities are to be undertaken to serve the objective of " ... improving the standard of service to the public of the building industry ...".

Our second starting point was the Pilot Study. This appreciation saw the primary source of the Industry's communications difficulties in the lack of relationship between the technical, economic and social forces now acting on and within the Industry, and the traditional resource controller roles, which between them are responsible for controlling the building process. Society's methods of financing its buildings and the size and time requirements of its demands on the Industry have all changed significantly in recent years. The rate of the Industry's development of its own techniques and materials has been equally remarkable, but the roles of those who jointly take responsibility for its operations have not developed similarly. The difficulties that are generated by this disparity in development show themselves in communications, the network of technical and social relationships forming the structure of the building team.

The basic requirement, therefore, seems to be a need for a conscious acceleration of the long process of adaptive evolution that various elements in the Industry have experienced, many of them over centuries, with the object of once more redefining them and their interrelationships to fit better the changing conditions in which they must now operate. This called for research of a kind that would allow the development of acceptable models for improving the efficiency of those who control resources. Improvement is needed, both in respect of the division of responsibility among them for the operations of the building process, as well as in respect of the patterns of relationship through which they work with each other for the common aim. The first requirement of such an undertaking is obviously a clarification of criteria for determining what are "improved" models.

The work of the Pilot Study had suggested two such criteria. The first is operational effectiveness. This obviously calls for a thorough operational knowledge of the building process to provide an objective technical datum for the whole pattern of interlocked operations involved. Such a study would need to be undertaken without regard to those traditional patterns in terms of which it is now usually conceived. Our second criterion was an appraisal of the economic, psychological and social possibilities and limits for change in the present resource-controller roles. This criterion would need to deal with the distinctive competence central to each of the existing resource-controller roles. From this analysis an appreciation could be made of the limits of possible change the present patterns of personal, professional and commercial commitments will allow without undue violence to any individuals or sections of the Industry. The work would also need to pay attention to society's functional and aesthetic needs in its buildings.

These considerations led us to the formulation of the next stage of the research. The establishment of a technical datum for the building process was to be undertaken by the application of the principles of operational research. This work should provide a basis for developing "ideal" models for the operations involved in the different phases of the process or parts of them. Only when the implications of these models have been modified by the findings under the second criterion will it be possible to make the practical suggestions which are our final objective. We all recognised that to achieve this result there would be need for much rigorous testing and modification to ensure that we got the basic models right.

We were aware that what we were suggesting was, of course, not entirely new. Consortia of professionals, client/design consortia, the builder's all-in service, negotiated contracts, etc., are all existing attempts to redefine in ways more appropriate to modern conditions the operational relationships between resource-controllers. What we are attempting to do is to provide a more comprehensive, more objective and more rational basis for such developments - in short to facilitate change.

When we came to tackle the problem of setting up a specific research programme in line with this general plan with the research team, our problem was one of rejection rather than selection. We had to set our aims within the constraints of our limited resources. Quite early we had to recognise that we could not attempt to tackle all aspects of the Building Industry, so we limited our work to the field of housing, the aspect thought to be most important for society at the present time. Within the field of housing we settled on three main phases of the building process to study in greater depth. The first is the briefing and design phase, the second the construction control phase, and the third a phase we have come to refer to as production planning, which covers all the activities between the designing operation and the construction of the building. It includes everything to do with costing and settling the tender, agreeing all aspects of the contract relationships, planning the construction, etc.

In each of these phases work is developing concurrently on operational model building as well as on the analysis of roles and their relationships. In each case the work is planned to proceed through three main stages: a first stage of observation leading to the setting up of a prototype model, a second stage of testing this model to establish a prima facie case for its soundness, and finally a stage of validation when we hope to have the developed model tried in real life situations. After only a year of work it is not yet possible to anticipate findings, but it is our hope that when the research is reported at the end of 1965 it will make a significant contribution to the development of our Building Industry.

THE UNIVERSITY,	JAMES OF RUSHOLME
YORK.	CHAIRMAN
December 1964	Building Industry Communications Research Committee

www.ingramcontent.com/pod-product-compliance
Lightning Source LLC
LaVergne TN
LVHW021112300926
849160LV00009B/705
* 9 7 8 0 4 1 5 4 8 4 1 5 2 *